*Claire's perseverance and determin[ation illustrate the] power of one individual's ability t[o heal when she] refused to accept prevailing medical wisdom. Her courage and dedication have inspired many others to pursue a path to health.*
Norman Schwartz, M.D.
Mequon, Wisconsin

*Claire is 100 percent right in concluding that food and/or chemical sensitivities are very important factors in many conditions. This, unfortunately, is not understood by specialists who should be experts.*
Marshall Mandell, M.D.
Bradenton, Florida

*When I, personally, applied the findings of Claire Musickant's research into the cause of fibromyalgia, I got my life back. This book, which results from her own experiences and studies, needed to be written so that other people who are needlessly suffering could be helped as I was.*
Elaine Gordon, Fibromyalgia Patient
Glendale, Wisconsin

*Claire Musickant has been an inspiration to me in my treatment of Fibromyalgia patients. Her persevering voice has provided an effective answer that has been largely ignored by traditional medicine.*
Michele Rozansky, Physical Therapist
Mequon, Wisconsin

*Perseverance is the pursuit of health and truth. That is what I learned from Claire Musickant in the time that I worked with her...and she made me work! Thank you, Claire, for what you taught me and will be sharing with others.*
Frank Fantazzi, Physical Therapist,
Orthopedic Certified Specialist
Milwaukee, Wisconsin

*Claire Musickant took a path that many fear to follow because of the barriers imposed by our current health care system. She fought the system and won her health through courage and decisiveness.*
Patricia A. Deuster, Ph.D., Master of Public Health
Bethesda, Maryland

*As a massage therapist, reading Claire's book has given me great insight and more tools to help me educate my clients. She takes readers through her own profound journey and her experience dealing with fibromyalgia. Best of all, she leads us to a place of incredible healing.*
Nancy Brittan, Massage Therapist
Wauwatosa, Wisconsin

*Three years ago I was afraid to walk the forty feet of our driveway to our mailbox for fear that I wouldn't have the energy to walk back to the house. It was very difficult for me to concentrate even long enough to read a page of a book. I would highlight sentences and not remember that I had read them. After two years of strictly following the guidelines that Claire presents in this book, and working with a nutritionist, acupucuturist and chiropractor, I regained my memory and physical strength so that I am actively working and now have the energy I had 20 years ago.*
Laurie Aleksandrowicz, Personal Financial Advisor
Franklin, Wisconsin

# FIBROMYALGIA:
## My Journey To Wellness

Claire Musickant

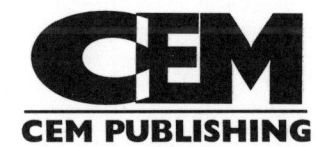

**CEM**
**CEM PUBLISHING**

Copyright © 1999, 2000, 2001 Claire Musickant

All rights reserved.

Cover Design by Mark Koerner
Text Design by Deb Lessila and Marc Daniloff

No part of this book may be reproduced or utilized in any form or by any means, electronic or mechanical, including photocopying and recording, or by any information storage and retrieval system, without permission in writing from the author.

ISBN 0-9639752-1-8
Library of Congress Catalog Card Number: 99-64037

First Printing November 1999
Second Printing 2001
Printed in the United States of America

Published by CEM Publishing
Milwaukee, Wisconsin

C E M   P U B L I S H I N G
P.O. Box 240035, Milwaukee, Wisconsin 53224

*In loving memory of*
*Pamela Rose Musickant and Randi Becker Glass*

# Acknowledgements

With joy and gratitude I thank all of the special people mentioned in this book who made this project possible, particularly the medical professionals who helped me get well; the study participants who supported the causal relationship between food and chemical sensitivities and their fibromyalgia symptoms; and all the many others who have shared their personal stories with me.

I also thank Edith Brin, whose work in reshaping my manuscript-in-progress was invaluable, Vera Hammerle for her cheerful support and her many computerized manuscript revisions, and Mark Koerner for his creative cover design. I would especially like to thank my husband Joseph Becker and our children and their spouses, who patiently (and sometimes not so patiently) listened to my tales of frustration and success.

# Table of Contents

**Introduction** ................................................................. i

## *Part I – There Must Be An Answer*

**Chapter 1 —**
1991: Hitting A Low Point ................................................. 1

**Chapter 2 —**
Getting To Know Me.......................................................... 7

**Chapter 3 —**
1984 To 1988: Onset & Progression ................................. 15

**Chapter 4 —**
1989: Diagnosis At Last .................................................... 23

## *Part II – The Mystery*

**Chapter 5 —**
1990: Going Downhill Fast ............................................... 35

**Chapter 6 —**
Learning About Fibromyalgia ........................................... 43

**Chapter 7 —**
Searching For Knowledge: The Diagnosis Dilemma .......... 57

**Chapter 8 —**
Searching For Knowledge: The Treatment Dilemma ......... 65

## Part III – Getting On With Life

**Chapter 9 —**
1991: Hope On The Horizon .................................................. 75

**Chapter 10 —**
1991: This Is A Remedy? ..................................................... 87

**Chapter 11 —**
1991: Learning About Sulfites & Other
Hazards To My Health ...................................................... 95

**Chapter 12 —**
1992: Expanding My Fibromyalgia Circle ...................... 103

## Part IV – Spreading The Word

**Chapter 13 —**
1992 - 1993: Calling In The Experts ............................... 111

**Chapter 14 —**
1994: Moving Forward ...................................................... 127

**Chapter 15 —**
The Stories Of Others ....................................................... 141

**Chapter 16 —**
1995: Complications ......................................................... 157

**Chapter 17 —**
1996: Results To Take Us To The Future ....................... 167

**Chapter 18 —**
How Can You Begin? ........................................................ 173

**Chapter 19 —**
My Life Today .................................................................... 185

**Epilogue 2001** ................................................................. 193

## *Appendices, Resources, & References*

**Appendix A —**
Comprehensive List of Items Tested ................................ 201

**Appendix B —**
ELISA/ACT™ Lymphocyte Response
Tests (complete) ............................................................ 207

**Appendix C —**
Description of Items Tested: Dairy Foods ........................ 210

**Appendix D —**
Symptoms or Conditions ............................................... 213

**Resources & References** .................................................... 214

# Introduction

I am a canary.

Canaries, as you probably know, are small birds, famous for their singing. They are usually yellow, but some are greenish, bluish, or any mixture of colors. They were first brought to Europe 500 years ago from the Canary and Madeira Islands, northwest of Africa. They eat seeds, live happily in cages for as long as 15 years, and become very fond of their owners.

I am not that kind of canary.

In recent history canaries also performed another kind of role, other than a happy seed-eating songster. In the early mining days, before mechanized devices were created, these caged singers were taken into the coal mines as early warning signals of the build-up of toxic and combustible fumes. When the canary keeled over, it was time to get out — fast.

Along with millions of others who have been diagnosed with Fibromyalgia Syndrome (FMS), Chronic Fatigue Syndrome (CFS), and Multiple Chemical Sensitivities (MCS), I am playing the role of the early-warning canary in our society. These syndromes (among many other autoimmune conditions) are indications that the ability of our immune system to protect us from the toxic pollutants in the air we breathe, the food we eat, and the water we drink is greatly reduced. While these conditions were essentially unheard of before the 1940s and are still exceedingly rare in indigenous cultures, they have become increasingly prominent within the last 30 years.

> These immune responses reflect an 'experiment' in which we participate by living in a rapidly restructured society (often without having signed an informed consent) affecting our food supply, our family relationships and our psychological expectations. This pace of adaptive change has accelerated in the last 40 years, a remarkably short time for biologic adaptation and learning of coping skills.[1]

My story is the story of many of us with the syndrome known as fibromyalgia. The average time between onset of symptoms and diagnosis is five years. Most of the information provided to us falls into the category of coping. We are told, "There is no cure."

To date, I continue to read the most current information from those actively promoting the "coping" route. I attend conferences, public forums, and lectures on fibromyalgia offered at local hospitals, clinics, or other locations. What is clearly obvious is that the standard medical therapies of prescription medication, and the self-help therapies such as relaxation, low-level exercise, deep breathing, stretching, and water therapy appear to be our only options.

More encouraging, however, is a recent, timid approach to the subject of nutrition by the medical community in relation to these syndromes. A healthy diet is frequently recommended, with an emphasis on potatoes, rice, pasta, fresh fruits, vegetables, and light meats (such as chicken and fish), along with avoidance of substances such as caffeine, alcohol, artificial sweeteners, sugar, and tobacco. Reluctant suggestions are also made to take multi-vitamins and other nutritional supplements.

More than 2,000 years ago, Hippocrates, the father of medicine, wrote:

> ...it appears to me necessary to every physician to be skilled in nature, and to strive to know, if he would wish to perform his duties, what man is in relation to the articles of food and drink, and to his other occupations, and what are the effects of each of them to everyone.[2]

I have written this book to let you know there is hope for a long-term, lasting cessation of all symptoms of fibromyalgia and that there is wellness — the defense and repair of our autoimmune systems. This state of wellness need not be a remission, but a continuing state of health and feeling of well being.

---

[1] Russell Jaffe, M.D., Ph.D. Immune Defense and Repair Systems in Biologic Medicine I: Autoimmunity, Clinical Relevance of Biological Modifiers in Diagnosis, Treatment and Testing.

[2] McCarrison, R. Nutrition and Health (London: Faber, 1964)

# Part I

## THERE MUST BE AN ANSWER

# Chapter 1
## 1991: HITTING A LOW POINT

*Bad times have a scientific value.*
*These are occasions a good learner would not miss.*
— EMERSON, *CONDUCT OF LIFE: CONSIDERATIONS BY THE WAY*

It was late morning on a bright summer day in 1991 as I sat at the desk in my study. I was fond of this cozy room, with its cushioned sofas and crammed bookshelves. My reference books were here, and what I call my "rest-your-head" reading. Alongside the books were photo albums filled with happy memories of family and travels.

This condominium in Glendale, Wisconsin, a northern suburb of Milwaukee, had been my home since my second marriage, almost nine years ago.

On this morning I was attempting to write some letters, pay some bills, and make some phone calls. My thoughts, however, were distracted. Despite the beautiful day and the comfort of my home, I was feeling anxious, depressed, angry, fatigued, and, most of all, impatient.

Impatient not only with my illness but with the medical profession as well. For not only was it not helping me with my physical problems, but in many cases, it was adding its own level of frustration.

My symptoms were becoming worse. Tender points (the defining criteria of fibromyalgia) along with tight muscles in my neck, back, arms and legs were causing me unbearable pain.

To compound the problems, I also had a collection of other symptoms numerous enough to comprise a medical dictionary in themselves. The details would sound ridiculous if they weren't describing my relentless agony.

I had alternating diarrhea and constipation (irritable bowel syndrome), headaches unrelieved by aspirin, unremitting fatigue, periodic allergy-like symptoms of swelling in my hands, itchy scalp and thinning hair, bleeding gums, photophobia (my eyes were abnormally sensitive to light), and temporomandibular joint (TMJ) pain on the left side of my face.

Is it any wonder I felt anxious and depressed and had trouble thinking and concentrating?

For more than seven years I had been living with these debilitating symptoms. They seemed to be gradually consuming my very existence. For the last two of those years I had the diagnosis of fibromyalgia. That was no help at all. According to my doctors, there was "No known cause and no known cure."

Fibromyalgia has been well described by the medical community since the mid-1800s. However, little attention was paid to this painful musculoskeletal condition until the 1980s. Often diagnosed by the absence of positive responses to tests for other disorders, fibromyalgia is commonly identified by a collection of symptoms, the most prominent of which is "tender points." The locations of these tender points are the same for all people with fibromyalgia, but not all fibromyalgia patients will have pain at all of the tender points. To be diagnosed with fibromyalgia, one must have pain associated with at least 11 of the 18 accepted locations. (See Figure 1.)

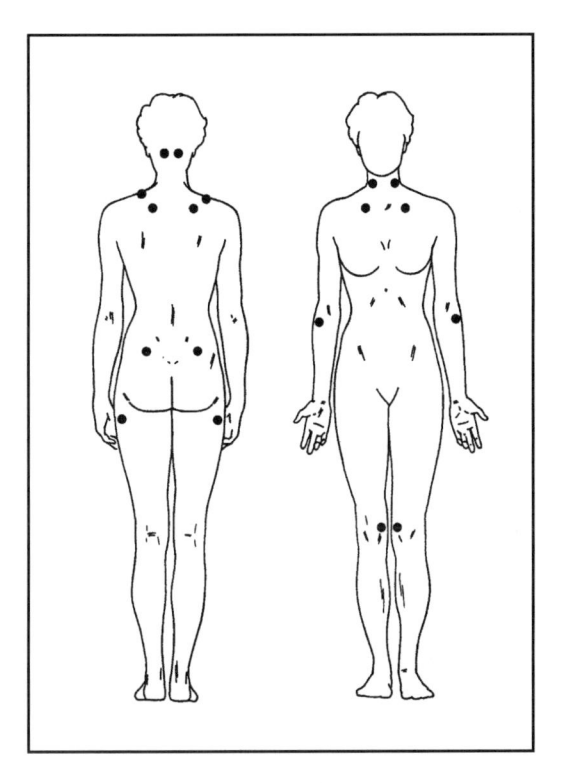

Figure 1. Tender Points

"Tender" is not always an accurate description. Sometimes these points, when pressed, can be excruciatingly painful. The pain of fibromyalgia is widespread: above the waist, below the waist, on the right side of the body and the left, up the spine, and through the chest. It must be consistently present for more than three months to be diagnosed as fibromyalgia.

Along with tender points and pain, fibromyalgia patients often suffer overwhelming fatigue.

As I would later learn, in 1993 the medical community began looking at the overlap between chronic fatigue syndrome and fibromyalgia syndrome. Sometimes it is difficult to distinguish between the two, so the diagnosis may be based on which is more pronounced, the pain or the fatigue (or with which condition the diagnosing physician is more familiar).

To further complicate the diagnosis and treatment of fibromyalgia, other conditions often occur at the same time. They include allergies, dry eyes and mouth, hair loss, irritable bowel syndrome, migraine-like headaches, premenstrual syndrome (PMS), muscle stiffness, vision changes, anxiety and depression, memory and concentration difficulties, and sleep problems, among others.

Not all fibromyalgia patients have all of these symptoms, but most have at least some of them. None of these symptoms, singly or collectively, is fatal, but at times many fibromyalgia patients wish they were.

My first response to receiving the diagnosis in 1989 was a feeling of hope. The symptoms had a name!

The phrase "No known cause, no known cure" didn't dampen that hope. In fact, it was more like waving a red flag in the face of an enraged bull. No way, I thought, was I going to accept this condition without a fight.

But here I was, two years later, unable to think clearly, needing to expend tremendous effort to perform the simplest tasks. Writing a check or a letter, making a phone call, completing any kind of paperwork, or sometimes just reaching for a pen, required more energy than I could summon. I had to fight for my sanity, for my physical health, and, most of all, for the quality of my life.

On that sunny summer morning after eating my usual breakfast of orange juice, scrambled eggs, toast with jelly and margarine, and a cup of coffee, my stomach started to churn and roil like a white-water river.

(It was much later I learned that nearly everything I had eaten that morning was taking its toll on my health.)

My thoughts turned to some of my friends, older than I, who still made dinner parties, played golf and cards, and visited friends and family with far more energy and enthusiasm than I could muster. I marveled at – and envied – their ability simply to make lunch for our Mah Jongg group, to smile, to entertain.

For the first two years following my diagnosis, I did everything the doctors recommended. But my physical condition was getting worse. Only 58 years old, I felt like Methuselah. The Bible says he lived 969 years, and I felt I was at about 960.

In spite of all of this, I managed to maintain a part-time career as an employee development consultant, educated myself about this strange and mysterious disease that had afflicted me, and continued to seek medical answers to my health problems.

The depression, however, was overwhelming. If this was what the rest of my life would be like, I wanted to slit my wrists. Fibromyalgia may not be life threatening, but at this point, it didn't matter. The quality of my life was rapidly slipping away.

# Chapter 2
## GETTING TO KNOW ME

*Adversity is the first path to truth.*
— BYRON, *DON JUAN CANTO XII, ST 50*

Adversity wasn't new to me. I grew up in the public housing projects of northwest Milwaukee. The brick barrack-like buildings were across the street from private homes that I now know were modest dwellings in a working-class neighborhood. But then they seemed to me like beautiful mansions. How wealthy those people must be, I thought, as I walked the seven blocks to school every day.

My parents had owned a small grocery store, but they lost it during the Depression. Following this loss, my father became clinically depressed, and eventually, when I was two years old, he required long-term hospitalization. He was released when I was ten. Until that time, I remember going to visit him only once. After his release, he did not live with my mother again until I had married and left home. My mother, brother, and I were supported by the welfare system.

It was adversity that molded and shaped me into a survivor. Beyond our economic and familial hardships, it wasn't particularly safe to be a Jewish girl growing up in those pre-World War II days. The community had a large German population and an active pro-Nazi German-American organization. Being Jewish meant being different and seemed to mean being inferior. I was chased home from grade school many times, called a "dirty Jew," and beaten up. The kindness of a boy named Glenn, who frequently walked me home from school to protect me, taught me that strength could also be gentle.

Even as a child, I found inner resources to give me strength. When life was difficult, I turned to books. The library was my refuge and my escape. From Jack London's *Call of the Wild* I learned lessons in perseverance and determination that are still part of who I am.

My parents' attitude about education was "boys go to college, girls go to work." This colored my feelings about school. Even though teachers tried to encourage my potential, my thinking was, "Why bother?" They urged me to take more academic courses on a college-bound track, but I was too ashamed and hurt to tell them there wouldn't be any money for college. (My brother, however, was encouraged to attend college and was supported while he earned his Ph.D. in biochemistry.) Instead I enrolled in commercial courses – typing, shorthand, bookkeeping – hoping to find a job after high school. And I was bored.

Having earned almost enough credits for high school graduation prior to my senior year, I attended classes only in the mornings and worked as a secretary for a nutritional supplement firm in the afternoons. One of the job perks was complimentary vitamins. After several months of this vitamin regimen, I seemed to have increased pep and energy.

What an interesting coincidence.

Shortly after graduation, while having lunch at a restaurant counter, a man sitting next to me started a conversation. No, this was not a Hollywood agent offering me stardom, the fantasy of every girl of my generation. But his offer seemed the next best thing – a full-time secretarial position in an insurance office with an increased salary of $35 per week.

Six months later, on a blind date, I met my future husband, Donald.

It was 1951 and the world was slowly recovering from the devastation of World War II. The face of the cityscapes was changing. With affordable housing for the returning servicemen springing up all over, there was a great sense of optimism and a belief in a never-ending peace. I was in love with Frank Sinatra, and even attended one of his performances. I never understood the squealing and screaming though. Mine was just a quiet adoration.

My cousin had told Donald about me. When he called to ask me out to a veteran's social, Donald said he was a graduate of my high school. I looked up his picture in the yearbook and decided he was good looking enough. I would accept.

The marriage, however...From flowers and poetry and constant attention, his behavior quickly turned into constant verbal and occasional physical abuse. My self-esteem plummeted.

I continued to work at the insurance company until the birth of our first child, Pamela. Then I helped by doing Donald's office work at home. We had four wonderful children – two daughters, Pamela and Cynthia, and two sons, Phillip and Daniel.

I had few marketable skills, and I chose to stay in the marriage to give our children the financial advantages of a suburban lifestyle and a college education. I stayed with Donald for 27 years, until my youngest child graduated from high school.

As my children matured and the pressures of raising my family ebbed, I turned my focus on myself. I sought help from a psychiatrist who encouraged me to enroll in college. I took some accounting, psychology, and speech courses at the local university. Then I took a short course in Transactional Analysis (TA). This tool for understanding myself and others so captured my interest that I underwent training to teach Transactional Analysis. The examining board of the International Transactional Analysis Association encouraged me to complete my college degree.

With a newfound courage, I pursued a B.A. in Management, got a part-time position teaching Transactional Analysis and Assertiveness, and filed for divorce. I was 47, and my life was taking flight with exciting new possibilities and challenges.

After my youngest child, Daniel, left for college, I moved into my own apartment. For the first time in my life I was living alone. Independence is not as easy or romantic as it sounds. I missed the energy of the children, the tumult of active family living, even the dog's affectionate attentions. Friends helped a little. I called one each evening, trying to fill the emptiness.

I also enrolled at Alverno, a local college to study business management. The college was starting an innovative program called "Competency-based Learning." This was a new concept that eliminated grades, but required written reports, public speaking, and group interactions, not just test results – to demonstrate the student's understanding of a particular subject.

After having attended a university with large "pit" classes, teaching assistants, and instruction via video instead of professors, I craved a more intimate learning environment. In this program the classes were small and taught by professors. They were even available for casual contact over lunch in the cafeteria or in the halls.

But it was the first year of the program, and there were plenty of glitches. Many days I felt like Alice in Wonderland looking for the Mad Hatter.

Still the months flew by as I attended classes, studied, worked part-time, and socialized with new and old friends. My son Daniel lived with me the following summer and provided the connection I'd been missing.

In June of 1981, my younger daughter, Cynthia, got married. It was a lovely, if somewhat modest, synagogue wedding with a luncheon reception in a downtown hotel. Cynthia, a petite size two, was stunning in the simple gown she had made herself. My ex-husband was there, and we were civil enough to each other, although we kept our distance.

That summer my older daughter, Pamela, lived with me. She was between semesters and working on her master's degree in science, hoping to become a nurse practitioner. She was also very health conscious and noticed that I was overweight and lacked energy. She started me on a regimen of daily morning walks – two miles in forty minutes. With a promise of orange juice, cottage cheese, bananas, and whole wheat toast – even occasionally eggs – waiting for me, I stuck with it. I began to feel wonderful, and I shed a few pounds too.

At the time, I was taking math courses in algebra and geometry toward my degree.

My life was about to take another of its sharp turns. One day Janet, a married friend, mentioned she had had someone named Joseph over for dinner several times since his wife died.

"What," I said. "You know a single man and didn't tell me!"

"He's too old," she said.

"Oh? Tell me more."

Well, it seemed this Joseph had a great sense of humor and was only 13 years older than I.

"I want to meet him," I said.

Janet and her husband invited Joseph and me to join them for dinner.

The chemistry was right. We talked, dated, got to know one another.

I liked his sense of humor. He doesn't tell jokes, but just finds life amusing. He's a good storyteller and has the ability to turn a clever phrase that makes people respond. He's a good listener, too.

Eventually we met each other's children. He came to my graduation. On December 19, 1981, my 49th birthday, I was awarded my B.A. in Management. I knew in my heart this program had been the right choice for me. I felt knowledgeable and competent and ready to move ahead.

We married on Joseph's birthday, October 31, 1982 (so he could remember our wedding date, he said), fourteen months after we met. All seven of our children and several of their spouses celebrated with us.

Two years later, my symptoms began.

When I had received my B.A. in Management one of my long-range goals had been to become an in-house trainer for a corporation. But the best the job recruiters could offer was a secretarial position with a promise of "possible" promotion to the training department in the future. It was the tough economy of the early 80s, and training wasn't a high priority. I felt like I was back where I started, 30 years earlier.

Fortunately the Women's Development Center at Waukesha County Technical College, where I was working part-time, offered me a short-term project to develop a program for Displaced Homemakers (widows, divorcees, and women who had never been employed) to assist them in the transition to the workplace. I could certainly identify with that.

I was to develop a similar program for Spanish-speaking women. My program was accepted and published. My good fortune continued when a career counseling position opened in the Women's Development Center and I got the job.

Our programs, "Building Self-Esteem", "Career Planning", "Resume Writing", and "Interviewing" helped develop confident, potentially successful employees. There were many success stories. My job was intellectually and emotionally satisfying. Much of the information and many of the skills I taught were also catalysts for change in my own life.

The three years from 1981 to 1984 were a time of joy and contentment, something I had never known before.

Joseph and I also discovered the delights of travel. We spent our first long vacation in the Canary Islands in 1983, and went to Russia in 1984.

We wanted more time for such pleasures. Joseph retired

from his job as director of housing production for HUD and started his own business as a consultant to the housing industry, specializing in residential needs for the disabled and the elderly. Several years later, his son Kenneth joined him in the business.

In September of 1984, I began freelance work as an employee development consultant for a management consulting firm, Measurable Performance Systems, Inc.

We did have more time to travel. But working on my own, I began to feel isolated. And I was struggling to sort out the insidious changes in my health from the emotional changes of being independently employed.

# Chapter 3
# 1984 TO 1988: ONSET & PROGRESSION

*O health! Health! The blessing of the rich! The riches of the poor! Who can buy thee at too dear a rate, since there is no enjoying this world without thee?*
— BEN JOHNSON, *VOLPONE* ACT II, SC. I

My very first effort to confront my health problem led to a diagnosis of food sensitivities. The results of that test, however, were not broad enough and missed the major contributors. It would take seven years of distress to finally confirm this.

Back then I visited the local wellness clinic, and they gave me a food sensitivity test for 195 allergens. When the test results came back, the nutritionist recommended that I eliminate various foods from my diet: dairy products, baker's yeast, avocado, beef, potatoes, spinach, black tea, MSG and saccharine, and all foods containing yeast, sugar, alcohol, or vinegar.

It sounded like a pretty drastic regimen, but there was even more. The nutritionist also recommended that I practice an elimination/four-day rotation diet, which means to eliminate all foods to which I am sensitive, and to eat other foods no more than once every fourth day. She prescribed a number of nutritional supplements to regulate my digestive system.

In retrospect, I realized I had significantly changed my eating habits in the previous five years, between 1979 and 1984. I had been living alone until 1982, had returned to college, and was working part-time. I was eating lunches and dinners at one school or the other, or in restaurants. Before 1979, I had done most of my own cooking. These dietary changes, I later learned, were overloading my immune system.

This prescribed wellness approach also emphasized the value of exercise. In addition to my daily 30-to 40-minute walk, I was encouraged to take a water aerobics class three to five times a week.

Following the new regimen, I initially felt better. I had fewer digestive problems and lost five pounds. I diligently followed the diet restrictions. Having achieved some measure of success, I adhered to the elimination and rotation diet wholeheartedly. I tried new foods such as rice cakes instead of bread, ate yams instead of white potatoes, stopped eating beef and ate more chicken, turkey, lamb, and fish. I drank no alcoholic beverages and eliminated all foods with sugar, yeast, and vinegar.

However, there was a hitch. In the process of modifying my diet, I had made two major substitutions. First, I switched from eating regular sugared jams and jellies to an all-fruit, sugar-free product. Second, I replaced the vinegar with lemon juice concentrate in my salad dressings.

Lemon juice concentrate and all-fruit jams – the substitutions seemed harmless enough. What I didn't know then was that these two food products contain a high percentage of sulfites/metabisulfites. These preservatives are present in many foods we eat, especially those prepared in restaurants and cafeterias.

These substitutions in my diet were taking a toll. I thought blithely that I was working my way toward better health. Instead, I was beginning to feel worse. Later, I would learn through experience that sulfites/metabisulfites have a cumulative effect on how I feel.

Despite my symptoms, I hadn't had a complete physical examination since 1982. In November of 1985, I went to my internist for a comprehensive health evaluation. The exam included blood chemistry and chest x-rays.

I told the doctor of the problems I was having, but he didn't offer any insights into what might be causing my ongoing health difficulties. He indicated in his notes that I had been diagnosed with yeast and dairy sensitivities. He also noted that my weight was stable, that I had a good appetite, and was generally in good health.

Later, looking back over those records, I would wonder if it was me he examined. In the months and years to come, as I researched the medical mystery that was changing my life, I requested copies of my medical records from all of the practitioners who had examined or treated me since the onset of my symptoms in 1984. Before that, I had had only short-term, treatable problems and had gone as long as nine years between complete health exams.

The next year, 1986, with a pain in my left big toe and a slight lower backache, I returned to the same internist for what I thought might be gout. (Gout is a disease that is often characterized by arthritic-like joint pains. It can be definitively diagnosed by measuring the level of uric acid in the blood, which will be elevated in gout patients.) My uric acid level was normal, and the doctor's notes indicated generalized arthralgia, the medical term for neuralgic (nerve-related) pain in the joints.

He prescribed Motrin, a form of ibuprofen that relieves inflammation, swelling, and stiffness associated with arthritic joint pain. The Motrin did nothing to relieve the pain, but at least I had no side effects.

By that time, I was doing a fair amount of self-diagnosis, and wondered if my toe and back were hurting because of the high-heeled shoes I wore to work.

I had thought it important that I look professional and stylish in my job as an employee development consultant. I was running training programs for colleges, universities, corporations, and state agencies, always appearing in front of new audiences. But walking from my car to various buildings and offices while carrying a briefcase and training materials was strenuous. And unfortunately for my feet and back, I was vain and continued to wear inappropriate shoes.

Since the Motrin seemed not to be the answer, I went back to the wellness clinic. For two years I had been faithfully following their prescribed program: an elimination/four-day rotation diet, water aerobics, and walking two miles a day.

My symptoms, primarily the pain in different places in my body, however, were worsening and my energy level was on a downward slide.

The nutritionist recommended another blood chemistry

test. The results showed allergies that had not appeared on the previous test in 1984. The allergens now included: cocoa, coffee, cod, cola, oregano, shrimp, and sugar cane. She adjusted the recommended nutritional supplements and I continued the four-day rotation/elimination diet.

But as the weeks passed, instead of improving, I continued to feel worse.

In the fall of 1986, I entered a new phase of increased pain and discomfort. Even turning over in bed became excruciating. My hands were swollen when I awoke in the morning. Pain had now spread to my hips and lower back, and the fatigue was unbearable.

Although I was continuing to take care with my diet, it was doing no good. I often wondered what would happen if I stopped regarding the food restrictions altogether.

One painful experience from that time stands out in my memory. I was conducting a training program at a local college. As the evening progressed, the pains got worse and worse, spreading from my toe to my hip to my lower back. When the class ended, people left promptly but it took me a few minutes to pack up my things. I think I was the only one remaining in the building. As I walked to the elevator, I wasn't sure I was going to make it, I was in such agony. Slowly, slowly I hobbled to the elevator, out of the building, and to the parking lot. The pain was excruciating, bringing tears to my eyes. I thought of taking off my shoes, but the air and the pavement were very cold – it was mid-November. With one slow, painful, agonizing step after another, I inched my way to the lone car left in the dimly lit parking lot. Finally, after what seemed an eternity, I was in the driver's seat. I sat for a moment to collect myself, and began a slow, painful drive home.

---

My faith in the medical profession was dwindling, but what else could I do? I went back to my internist. Same old complaints: low backache, joint pain in my hands and feet. He took x-rays that showed abnormal curvature in the lower spine, but not much else.

Another trip to the nutritional therapist got me another adjusted nutritional supplement, advice to continue the rotation/elimination diet, and to call her if I had any questions.

All in all, hurting, hurting and seeking, seeking, but no help to be found.

---

Joseph and I had enough financial independence to take a long vacation in Florida every winter. In early 1987, we again went for a month to the sunny South. We walked every day for a mile or more on the sun-drenched beaches, and I swam regularly in the ocean or a pool. We relaxed, we rested, we had fun, we dined out. And my physical well-being improved. So I chalked up all of the symptoms that had been plaguing me to work stress and fatigue.

But I was kidding myself.

Three months after our return to Milwaukee, a steady increase in my symptoms again sent me to the internist. I had pain in my elbows, knees, and hips. Anacin every morning helped me start the day. But each new day brought dread of the pain that wouldn't go away.

The doctor drew blood for an antinuclear antibody (ANA) screening test to check for rheumatoid arthritis and systemic lupus erythematosus (SLE). The tests were negative.

He examined my hips, elbows, and ankles. This time he concluded I had arthritis. His notes, however, referred to the problem as "polymyalgia rheumatica," which simply means pains all over.

In my naiveté, I did not ask for details about what kind of arthritis he thought I had, or what this meant medically. Arthritis, that sounded okay, it seemed manageable to me. I recalled my mother always complaining of aches and pains and still managing to function, so I said, "I guess I can live with that."

He prescribed Naprosyn (naproxen), a pain reliever in the class of nonsteroidal anti-inflammatory drugs (NSAIDs).

With the prescription in hand, I once again felt encouraged that my problem was now under control. But once again, how wrong I was!

I took the Naprosyn as prescribed, but my pain escalated, especially at night. Again, I couldn't turn over in bed. I didn't have to fall asleep to experience nightmares; they were there as I lay in bed, wide-awake and hurting.

Naprosyn is prescribed to relieve mild to moderate pain and symptoms of osteoarthritis, rheumatoid arthritis, ankylosing spondylitis (an arthritis of the spine), tendinitis, bursitis, and sudden gout attacks. I have since learned that NSAIDs do nothing to relieve the discomfort of fibromyalgia, and in some cases, can exacerbate the pain.

Somebody suggested a chiropractor. Why not? Nothing

else was working. From July 1987 to November 1988, I saw a chiropractor at various intervals, beginning several times a week, then decreasing the visits to twice a week, twice a month, and bi-monthly treatments. The chiropractor recommended that I continue my daily walking routine, discontinue the water aerobics and swim laps instead. She also told me to stop wearing high-heeled shoes, and I did. (I haven't worn them since, and miss them not one bit.) There seemed to be some relief from the body pain, but my lethargy and fatigue gradually increased, along with irritability, depression, and the inability to control my weight. Sad to say, some of the chiropractic neck adjustments added to my discomfort.

# Chapter 4
## 1989: Diagnosis At Last

*Look to your health; and if you have it, praise God,
and value it next to a good conscience;
for health is the second blessing we mortals are capable of;
a blessing that money cannot buy.*
— Isaak Walton, *Compleat Angler*, Pt. I, Ch. 21

Our blended family of seven children seemed to be nicely settling down. By January 1988, I had another son- and daughter-in-law, three more grandchildren, and two more on the way.

Early in our marriage, we had established a ritual of monthly Sunday brunches at our home so that our children could get to know each other. At these brunches we celebrated birthdays, anniversaries, and holidays.

As the grandchildren arrived and joined the family, the brunches got more chaotic and joyful. The adults watched and played with the babies as they developed – the sitting up, the first teeth, the first steps. Because I always felt better during our winter vacations, Joseph and I decided to buy a condominium in Florida and to lengthen our time there in the future. We looked forward to having the families join us in

Florida. Everything seemed so right.

But then the sky fell in.

It was a weekend in July of 1988, and I had returned to our new condominium in Florida, in order to prepare it for our arrival in winter. We had purchased it fully furnished. When we first saw it, I knew it was the right place for us – it felt homey. It was carpeted in dark colors that could take casual living, the wear of little feet and sticky fingers. It had lots of windows and two balconies, one of which overlooked the swimming pool and an inland waterway. However, it needed a lot of "spit and polish." I happily dusted, vacuumed, and scrubbed in preparation for the good times to come – having our children join us the next winter.

On Sunday, feeling somewhat restless, I swam in the pool and briefly met some of our new neighbors. I went out for an early dinner and drove to the ocean, thinking the tranquillity of seeing the water and watching the waves rolling in would have a calming effect. I stayed for only a short time, sensing I needed to return to the condo. Still feeling agitated, I thought about going to a movie. Finding nothing of interest in any nearby theater, I settled for some TV watching.

Suddenly I was startled by the ringing of the doorbell. When I called, "Who's there?" a woman's voice responded, "Sheriff's Department."

I opened the door to find a short stocky woman dressed in a nondescript uniform. She curtly told me to call home. When I said I had no phone she said, "There's one across the street at the shopping center," then turned abruptly and left.

As I absorbed what she said, my body felt numb and in shock. I went down the elevator and ran across the street to the phone. Filled with dread, I dropped the coins in the slot and made a collect call.

When Joseph answered the phone, I knew he was okay, but I could hardly bear to hear his next words. As gently as possible, and making sure I understood, Joseph told me my older daughter, Pam, had been killed in a motorcycle accident. She and her husband, each on their own bike, were returning from a weekend of camping and visiting friends' children at a camp in central Wisconsin. My two-year-old grandson was at home with his other grandmother.

The numbness and shock intensified as Joseph and I talked about whether he should come to Florida to get me. No, I couldn't wait for him. I would try to get an early-morning flight.

Not knowing another soul in the area, I returned to the condo and rang the manager's bell. He and his wife were kind and invited me in to use their phone to make my flight arrangements.

I knew I wouldn't be able to sleep, so I packed my bags, closed up the condo and drove the rental car back to the airport. Along with several homeless people, who slept on the airport lounges, I sat from 2 A.M. until almost eight. The repetitious announcements on the loudspeakers – "watch your step on the escalators", "hold the hand of small children" – droned in my ears. Nothing penetrated my deadened senses. I sat and waited, frozen and unfeeling.

At the airport in Milwaukee, Joseph, Pam's husband Kris, and my grandson Ben were waiting. Ben didn't know yet. How do you tell a two year old that he will never see his mommy again?

We went to my daughter Cynthia's home where the rest of the family had gathered. We cried, consoled each other, and made the funeral arrangements.

I called a children's psychotherapist for advice about how to tell my grandson. She explained that it was important to be truthful. Ben needed to know his mommy was dead and how she died; and that he would never see her again. It was also important that he attend the funeral.

He did, and he placed a pink rose on her casket. Fortunately, Ben was very verbal and could talk about and understand what had happened. Several visits to the therapist helped him gain more understanding and acceptance.

I ignored my own feelings in trying to help our other children. It seemed to me that the most important thing was to be supportive of each other and to maintain the family closeness. My greatest fear was the disintegration of the family Joseph and I had nurtured and shaped so lovingly. Spending more time together and continuing the Sunday brunches eased our heartache. We also now had two more grandchildren, who were a reminder that it is important to appreciate the joys of life along with enduring the pain.

The magnitude of this disaster was so devastating that I abandoned all concerns about food, diets, and exercise. At this point it was hard to tell the physical aches and pains from the mental and emotional anguish.

A few visits to a psychotherapist were a little relief, although the only thing I remember him telling me more than once is that "sh*t happens." A woman whose daughter had recently died told me the pain never goes away.

I thought, If the pain lasts and is this bad, I will never make it. How does one get through this? For some, it means moving slowly; for me, nothing seemed to ease the numbness and shock except forcing myself to keep busy. And busy I stayed – working, spending time with my children and grandchildren, forcing myself to socialize, and retreating into escape literature.

When I was working, I could forget for an hour or two. I realized if I could do that, perhaps I would be able to survive.

The winter vacation time – now extended to two months – which we had looked forward to with such delight, was shaded by our loss, but four of our children and their families spent time with us. Again, a reminder that life does go on.

---

It had been nine months since Pam's death, and two months in Florida had not relieved my symptoms. It was time for another opinion.

I decided to look for a new internist and chose a woman, thinking she might be more sympathetic to my problems. It was more of the same – blood work, x-rays, etc. I lay on the cold, hard x-ray table feeling despair, twisted into positions for views I knew were unlikely to show anyone anything that hadn't been seen before.

As usual, all the tests were normal! "Then why do I have such excruciating pain?" I asked. The doctor seemed just as baffled.

Even though a test for arthritis symptoms was negative, she gave me a sample of Volteran. Volteran, generic name diclofenac sodium, is used to treat mild-to-moderate pain and symptoms of rheumatoid arthritis, osteoarthritis, and spondylitis. Diclofenac is an NSAID, the family of drugs often used to treat arthritis in older adults, although many believe that aspirin is just as effective and less costly.

I brought to my appointment an article about a condition called "fibromyalgia." The description of this condition, which I'd only vaguely heard of, sounded awfully close to home:

> [Fibromyalgia is] classified as a rheumatic disorder that can cause pain, tenderness and stiffness in muscles and tendons at specific "trigger points" that are distributed over the back of the neck and shoulders, the sides of the breast bone and the bony points of the elbows and hips. In addition, there are a whole flock of non-rheumatic symptoms to complicate the patient's life, including poor sleep, anxiety, fatigue, and even irritable bowel symptoms.
> 
> (Bruckheim 1988)

The doctor ignored the article and dismissed this idea with a wave of her hand. She prescribed Halcion, a sleeping pill that has had a great deal of negative press. I had heard that Halcion should be avoided by older adults because it is so short-acting it can cause rebound insomnia, anxiety, forgetfulness or memory loss, and violent aggressive behavior. I elected not to fill the prescription. However, that evening I did take one Voltaren, and I awoke in the morning with a headache beyond description. When I called the doctor to tell her about this reaction, she said, "Wait a day and try it again." No way! I was not interested in the risk of experiencing that kind of excruciating pain again.

I felt the doctors were just experimenting, prescribing whatever sample the latest pharmaceutical representative happened to leave behind, without any definitive reason for the prescription. I wasn't keen about being a guinea pig, but I wasn't ready to give up on the medical profession either. I got copies of my x-rays from the radiologist and started making the rounds of other medical disciplines.

I tried an orthopedist. Another dead-end.

Not everything in his report was even accurate. I was beginning to detect a pattern of doctors not really paying attention to what I was telling them.

After the examination he said he needed to do some further tests. When I asked what this might entail, in a spooky voice he responded, "We will need to do a myelogram."

I declined. It seemed to me he was "fishing," and I didn't need that. I hadn't learned what was wrong with me, but I was learning a little about navigating the unreliable waters of the medical system.

My pain and fatigue continued to increase, now by leaps and bounds. In desperation, I sought out another chiropractor. This one examined the x-rays and was a little more honest. He said if he couldn't help me in 10 visits, then I should search for some other kind of help.

For six weeks I went to each treatment with hope and optimism. Each time I would feel better, but only briefly. Sometimes the pain relief would last for a day or two, but more often by the time I arrived home, the pain was back, and sometimes worse.

Then one day, my daughter Cynthia gave me the name of a new doctor, an internist who also practices homeopathic medicine. (Homeopathy is a holistic approach that uses small amounts of natural substances to stimulate the body's own healing power.)

I liked the idea of seeing someone who might look at my symptoms in a different context. With x-rays in hand, I went to Dr. Anthony Sweeney for yet another opinion. I've lost count of how many I'd had so far.

I remember the day clearly. It was a glorious early summer day with warm sun, balmy breezes, and a vividly blue, almost cloudless sky. Considering how I was feeling, it's a wonder I continued going from one doctor to another, ever hopeful. Where was that hope coming from? There certainly hadn't been much to sustain it lately.

The casual style of other doctors had made me suspicious and distrustful. The doctors had acted as if they knew the answers while hardly even listening to the questions. They seemed to give no careful thought or consideration to my symptoms, or even to the x-rays and tests that had been done by my growing list of doctors. I'm sure some dismissed me as a hypochondriac or in need of psychiatric help. As I now know, if a practitioner is unfamiliar with fibromyalgia, a patient can be easily dismissed with a diagnosis of mental dysfunction.

It's funny how at the gut level we can feel immediately when something is right.

My first visit with Dr. Sweeney began in a wonderfully heartening way. At last I had found a physician who listened! While I sat on the examining table, Dr. Sweeney looked at the x-rays, took a medical history, and paid attention as I described where the pain was.

He checked some points in my back, the front of my knees, and my elbows. After the examination, he asked me to come into his office. I eagerly awaited what he had to say. He told me I had myofascial pain syndrome, also known as fibromyalgia.

At last! A diagnosis! A word to describe what I was living with! I was so excited that my condition finally had a name.

"So what do we do about this?" I naively asked.

Dr. Sweeney answered with words I didn't want to hear

and refused to accept. "There is no known cause and no known cure."

He did offer that some patients feel relief by taking Barley Green, a nutritional supplement. He also recommended that I see an osteopath.

I liked that idea. Osteopathy is the school of medicine that believes the body is a machine that, when properly adjusted, can produce its own remedies against infections and other disabling conditions. It focuses on the relationship of the musculoskeletal system to the other systems, and since much of my misery was musculoskeletal, it made sense to me. I made an appointment with Allan Robertson, a Milwaukee doctor of osteopathy.

Dr. Robertson is a gentle, empathic clinician; another doctor who finally listened attentively to my description of symptoms. Later he would tell me fibromyalgia is one of the most resistant, least-rewarding conditions you can treat. He said he has seen fibromyalgia present in a variety of ways, spent years nailing down a diagnosis for some patients, and found the response to treatment very elusive. He was very sympathetic to the "doctors-be-damned" attitude I was rapidly developing.

At the start of his examination, he asked me to stand straight but comfortably, with my arms at my sides. He then asked me to look over my shoulder into the mirror. I didn't like what I saw. What I thought was a comfortably erect posture was anything but. My head stuck out like a turtle peering out of its shell. My back was bent over, and my ribs were close to touching my belly, with no waistline between.

While I sat on the therapy table, Dr. Robertson asked me to turn my head, first to the right, and then to the left. My response was pretty feeble; first a shift of my eyes in the requested direction, followed by a partial turn of my head.

Dr. Robertson proceeded to work on realigning my posture and relieving the tightness of the muscles, especially in relation to the tender points. Starting with my lower back and hips, he worked the muscles that were taut and instructed me about stretching exercises to work on at home.

I continued this therapy once or twice a week, as I felt the need, and faithfully performed the exercises at home daily.

In August, about a month after my first visit, I returned to Dr. Sweeney. He suggested I try Arnica, a homeopathic remedy. It gave me a headache.

I asked him if it were possible that food sensitivities had anything to do with my poor health. I mentioned milk and severe sugar cravings. He noted the question in my medical records, but he didn't pursue the idea.

I continued the therapy, the exercises at home, and the Barley Green, which I found at a local health food store. This approach helped me cope with the pain, and it seemed to diminish somewhat. However, I was still struggling with fatigue and other symptoms that were not severe as yet.

Before Joseph and I left for our winter break in Florida, Dr. Robertson suggested I learn to swim the backstroke and continue the daily stretching exercises at home. The backstroke helps keep the back muscles aligned and stretches the chest muscles at the same time.

I still didn't share with Joseph, my children, or anyone else the extent of the ever-increasing pain and fatigue I was experiencing. With everything I was trying to do to relieve these symptoms, I couldn't believe they were going to persist and become an incessant part of my life.

# Part II

## The Mystery

# Chapter 5
# 1990: Going Downhill Fast

*The preservation of health is a duty. Few seem conscious that there is such a thing as physical morality.*
— Herbert Spencer, *Education*, Ch. 4

We had been in Florida for two months, and it was only a few days before we were to return to Wisconsin when I ate that unforgettable pizza. Next thing I knew, I was in a hospital emergency room with such intense pain in my face that it felt like the bones were going to break apart.

When I finally got to an examining room, the doctor seemed bewildered that I could have such pain without any apparent physical cause, although my temperature was slightly elevated. When I told him I was returning north in a few days and would see my own physician, he prescribed a sinus medication to carry me over until then. I couldn't take the medication because it made me drowsy; we were driving home, and I needed to take my turn at the wheel.

Once back in Milwaukee, I saw Dr. Sweeney, who had more to add to my ever-proliferating medical records: the facial pain, the 100-degree temperature, a dry cough, and a burning sensation at the back of my tongue. He prescribed Natur-Muir (another homeopathic remedy). He also noted in my medical records that my fibromyalgia was gone.

He may have thought the fibromyalgia was gone, but I was not quite so optimistic. The Natur-Muir was masking some of the symptoms, but it didn't last. Two weeks later the fibromyalgia symptoms – pain, fatigue, and headaches – were back with a vengeance.

The next 18 months were a constant round of visits to Dr. Robertson for body work and to Dr. Sweeney for further trials of Natur-Muir. At times, this remedy seemed to help, but gradually my body began to feel like an automobile parked in neutral, with its motor revved at great speed. My internal motor was racing, but my body couldn't move.

During this time I had pain, a runny nose, and itchy, watery eyes. Some days I felt great, but more often I was plagued by respiratory symptoms: itching in my throat, laryngitis, and a persistent cough. There were also many days of fatigue, depression, and anxiety when all I wanted to do was curl up in a fetal position and shut out the world.

My visits to Dr. Robertson resulted in only temporary relief of my body pain. More and more of my time was spent in walking, stretching exercises, and swimming. I felt as if I had no life but the time-consuming efforts of trying to keep my body going. The rest of the time I was debilitated by the fatigue and depression.

Working had become more and more difficult. I tried rescheduling some of my training programs into two half-day programs instead of full day-long programs. I frequently needed a chair to lean against or hold onto, sometimes resting one knee on the seat to relieve the pain. Each day of work was usually followed by a day or two of fatigue and resting, forcing me to schedule training days less and less frequently. I still enjoyed my classes, but the pain involved was giving me mixed feelings about my work. I came to dread the phone calls requesting my services.

The only thing that distracted me from my misery during this time was an insatiable need to better understand fibromyalgia, the "mystery syndrome."

Where to start? I called some of the teaching hospitals in the Milwaukee area to see if I could use their libraries. I started with the Columbia Hospital Medical Library. The librarian graciously gathered information from various books and journals for me. Some of it was very technical and bewildering, but I applied myself.

The more I read, the less confusing the information became. Some articles had summaries, which were written in a less technical manner. I had several of the articles copied. I was feeling optimistic .

I called the Arthritis Society, which sent me several booklets relating to fibromyalgia and arthritis in general. There was material being written, and that, in itself, was reassuring. But what I read was of little comfort. I subscribed to the *Fibromyalgia Network* newsletter and sent for a guide entitled *Coping With Fibromyalgia.* I gained more knowledge, but no encouragement that there was anything to do but cope. Coping did not sound promising.

The Hindus say, "Once you start looking, you can't stop seeing." When one has a medical condition, it's amazing how many people one meets who also have this problem.

I talked to women who attended fibromyalgia support

groups where, as they described it, most of the time was spent commiserating with each other and lamenting their state of health. Their major focus seemed to be petitioning the government for increased funds for research. One woman said her rheumatologist told her to take hot showers when the pain became unbearable. She would undress several times a day and do just that. This suggestion did not sound practical to me.

I was also told that a medical practitioner who spoke at one of these meetings suggested to the group that they go home and grieve over the loss of their health and the former healthy condition of their bodies. Grieving? Coping? That was not what I wanted. The very thought of spending the rest of my life this way was outrageous! I was angry at the diagnosis; angry at the amount of time I spent just walking, swimming, and stretching; angry enough to feel I could not let this continue. I wanted a life!

I decided I needed to learn more. I went to the Wisconsin Medical College Library. A kind librarian searched the computer for a seemingly endless list of articles focusing on various aspects of fibromyalgia. Armed with a list covering the history, diagnosis, possible causes, relation to other syndromes (such as chronic fatigue syndrome), onset, and treatment, I selected 30 articles that I felt I could read, digest, and understand. I made copies of the articles and went home to study.

I spent the summer of 1991 reading and organizing this information. It was encouraging to know that I was not alone, that many suffered the frustrating symptoms that had become the hallmark of my life, and that considerable scientific attention was being devoted to this subject. The research

I did that summer provided the foundation for the attack I launched on this disease.

---

Since the time of my diagnosis, I had been scouring the medical literature for whatever I could find about fibromyalgia. Though I was depressed and discouraged that summer morning two years after the diagnosis, I was not ready to give up hope.

At a medical library, I found a chapter from a rheumatology textbook on nutrition and rheumatic disease. It did not directly relate to fibromyalgia, but fibromyalgia is considered a rheumatic disease. I carefully re-read the chapter. Some passages rang a bell. Suddenly I sensed a real relevance. I read:

> Although there is little evidence at present that variations in diet have important effects on rheumatic diseases, experimental progress in this area suggests that we may be on the threshold of significant discoveries in understanding the role of nutrition in human health and disease in general, and in inflammatory rheumatic diseases in particular.
>
> ... it is now being recognized that ingestion of a food may result in clinical symptoms. Some examples are delayed – onset food sensitivity, chronic gastroenteropathy, and gluten-and milk-induced gastroenteropathy. (Briones and Robinson 1989)

The authors described a patient with rheumatoid arthritis whose disease was exacerbated by the ingestion of dairy products. Exclusion of dairy products from her diet produced a considerable improvement in her disease. Another report came from a dermatologist who concluded that his own recurring rheumatism was due to hypersensitivity to sodium nitrate, a preservative that is in many foods. Still another study found that some subjects reacted with rheumatic joint and muscle reactions after ingesting certain food extracts.

> These observations suggest that adverse reactions to food and environmental antigens can bring about rheumatic symptoms to predisposed individuals, the author suggested, concluding that the role of hypersensitivity in rheumatic diseases needed to be examined more carefully.(Briones and Robinson 1989)

It made a lot of sense to me as I thought of the progression of my symptoms.

I knew I needed to explore other treatment approaches. I sought out two other specialists. One was a physical therapist who uses a technique called myofascial release. The other was an internist who specialized in nutrition problems. Myofascial release is a manual therapy aimed at mobilizing, softening, and relaxing muscles and connective tissue. This allows muscle to sit in its normal position. With correct alignment between the skeleton and the muscle, it is then easier to strengthen the muscle.

Without consulting anyone, I simply picked up the phone and made appointments with both of them. (You might, however, need to get a referral from your doctor for insurance purposes.)

It was still a beautiful summer morning. It was also a day which would be the turning point on my journey of discovery and healing. Moreover, it would set me on the road to spreading the word that there is help and recovery from this mysterious syndrome that has engrossed my life and the lives of so many others.

# Chapter 6
# LEARNING ABOUT FIBROMYALGIA

*All our progress is an unfolding, like the vegetable bud. You first have an instinct, then an opinion, then a knowledge.*
— EMERSON, *ESSAYS, FIRST SERIES: INTELLECT*

Fibromyalgia (pronounced: fye-bro-my-AL-juh) is a disorder characterized by diffuse, widespread musculoskeletal aching and stiffness, multiple tender points, and non-restorative sleep (sleeping without feeling rested). In medical terminology, fibromyalgia is a syndrome rather than a disease. A syndrome is a collection of symptoms or combination of qualities that constitute a disorder, or a group of signs and symptoms that collectively indicate or distinguish a disease, psychological disorder, or other abnormal condition.

Syndromes are different from diseases. In the case of a syndrome like fibromyalgia, the symptoms tend to be very frustrating and very subtle. This syndrome does not kill people. It does not cause deformities or cosmetic problems, and is not degenerative. Because most patients with fibromyalgia look healthy, friends, family, and even many doctors fail to take their complaints seriously and may doubt that the pain and fatigue are real. Many times patients are told, "I can't find anything. Your blood tests are normal. Your x-rays are normal. Maybe it's all in your head. Go see a psychiatrist."

My own pattern, as I discovered in my research, is quite typical. Many other patients with fibromyalgia go through a succession of doctors before they finally get a diagnosis. On average, this takes five years. Dr. Kenneth Nies, a rheumatologist who practices in Torrence, California, and teaches at UCLA, points out that some physicians may not have heard of the "tender point" concept or various other indications of fibromyalgia. He says that since patients have often been told that their symptoms are all in their heads, and there is nothing physically wrong with them, it can be a great relief for them to find out they really do have a physical condition. Although fibromyalgia syndrome is included among the 100 or so different rheumatic diseases characterized by arthritis (which causes pain and swelling in the joints), fibromyalgia's pain is in the ligaments, tendons, and muscles. Yet, it can affect the way joints function.

Patterns of widespread musculoskeletal pain have been noted since the time of Hippocrates, but it has only been in the last 150 years that the diagnostic potential of musculoskeletal symptom clustering has been recognized.

In 1904, William Gowers, a British neurologist, coined the term "fibrositis," assuming that the symptoms he was observing were due to *inflammation* of the fibrous tissue. Dr. Gower's term was given further credibility when reports on biopsies showed inflammation in the fibrous tissue of patients who had reported muscular aching, stiffness, and fatigue.

However, these findings were never replicated, and "fibrositis" is a misleading label. The lack of any underlying inflammation in fibromyalgia has been confirmed by the observation that fibromyalgia patients do not respond to either corticosteroids or nonsteroidal anti-inflammatory drugs (NSAIDs).

*The 25th edition of Stedman's Medical Dictionary* (1995), the standard for the medical profession, still names this syndrome "fibrositis" and has no entry for "fibromyalgia." No wonder doctors are confused!

In the 1960s and 70s, researchers Smythe and Modolfsky noted the combined symptoms of chronic diffuse pain, nonrestorative sleep, and predictable tender points among some patients. They started to lay the groundwork for what has become a generally accepted criterion for fibromyalgia. Currently, fibromyalgia is the focus of a great deal of medical and scientific attention. In 1980, my search revealed that there was not one single reputable article about fibromyalgia in the entire world. In 1990, there were 175. There has been a real explosion of interest, not just in the U.S., but throughout the world, particularly in Scandinavian countries and England.

In the past decade or so, fibromyalgia syndrome has emerged from the realm of vague, controversial disorders. At one time, fibrositis was considered a label for any poorly understood chronic muscle pain or the existence of a psychiatric condition (referred to as psychogenic rheumatism). Today, fibromyalgia is a commonly offered and generally accepted diagnosis. Investigators have shown that patients with fibromyalgia have uniform symptoms and signs, thus demonstrating that the syndrome is a consistent entity.

It is typical for fibromyalgia patients to see many different physicians and try many therapies without much benefit. Most patients are sent to numerous specialists and undergo costly, and sometimes invasive, diagnostic tests that usually serve only to reinforce their fear that they harbor some undiscovered, dreaded illness. Psychiatric referrals are often helpful in terms of therapy that can help patients deal with their symptoms, but sometimes this leads to mistrust and anger directed against the medical profession. Who wants to be told that all their pain is only in their head?

Elderly patients who complain to their physicians about joint pain and stiffness may be showing signs of fibromyalgia as well as some other rheumatic condition. Failure to consider fibromyalgia as a possibility in elderly patients can lead to misdiagnosis and to over-treatment with corticosteroids or immunosuppressants for inactive rheumatoid arthritis, or to unnecessary investigations or surgery for back pain.

Fibromyalgia is neither fatal nor crippling. By the time patients are diagnosed, however, they are usually anxious, frustrated, depressed, angry, tired, and impatient with their illness and the medical profession.

To help family and friends relate to fibromyalgia, have them think back to the last time they had a bad flu. Every muscle in their body shouted out in pain. They may have felt completely lacking in energy, as though someone had unplugged their power supply. This pain and weakness is typical of fibromyalgia, as are a number of other symptoms.

Fibromyalgia could be termed "the great impostor," because its signature – diffuse musculoskeletal aches and pains associated with tender points – is mimicked by dozens of other medical conditions.

Fibromyalgia is so tricky to diagnose that frequently a precise diagnosis is made only by first ruling out what it is not. Often a variety of x-rays and blood tests are required to eliminate the possibility of diseases like Parkinson's or rheumatoid arthritis. Other syndromes associated with chronic generalized musculoskeletal pain, stiffness, and tenderness include: chronic fatigue, irritable bowel, and possibly postviral syndrome, and multiple chemical sensitivities.

Most investigators agree that there is a significant overlap between these syndromes and that they may be only parts of a more generalized condition that includes chronic headache, roving numbness, TMJ syndrome, and a host of other physical pain syndromes.

Chronic musculoskeletal pain syndromes are common problems, but the causes, development, and consequences of many of them are poorly understood. In spite of the prevalence of fibromyalgia symptoms, and the disrupting effects these symptoms have on sufferers' lives, the first detailed and controlled study of the clinical characteristics of fibromyalgia was not published until 1981.

## Epidemiology and Causes

Fibromyalgia appears to be a very common ailment. Although the extent of fibromyalgia is difficult to determine, current estimates suggest that one to four percent of Americans have the condition. The syndrome seems far more common among women than men, with women accounting for 80 to 95 percent of all fibromyalgia patients. It is unclear whether this pattern represents a difference in underlying physical mechanisms, a difference in the way that symptoms are reported, or the fact that women are more likely to seek medical care than men.

The onset of fibromyalgia usually occurs between the ages of 20 and 70, although some teenagers, and even younger children, have symptoms just as severe as their middle-aged and elderly counterparts. The age of medical presentation is considerably higher than age of onset, suggesting that the typical patient endures symptoms for a number of years before receiving an appropriate diagnosis.

The cause of fibromyalgia remains difficult to pinpoint, but there are many triggering events thought to cause its onset. Approximately 50 percent of patients associate a specific event with an abrupt onset of symptoms. The events include physical or emotional trauma, or an illness, such as a viral syndrome. On the other hand, some patients describe an insidious onset over a long period of time, which is what I experienced.

Many doctors find that sleep disturbance is a symptom common to all fibromyalgia patients and even speculate that this may be the underlying pathway leading to the syndrome. Types of sleep disturbances in fibromyalgia patients run the gamut: light sleepers, women with young children who awaken frequently during the night, patients with inflamed joints who can't find a comfortable position in bed, patients taking diuretics who awaken frequently to use the bathroom, patients who may awaken frequently to drink water, and patients who are married to a spouse who snores loudly.

An early theory about the cause of fibromyalgia attributed the syndrome to inflammation of the fibrous tissue, possibly due to the Epstein-Barré virus or other infectious agent. But there has been no consistent evidence of viral inflammation in the areas of tenderness, and the theory upholding an infectious cause has fallen from favor. Patients, however, still sometimes hold to this misconception. In a recent study, 55 percent of patients with fibromyalgia attributed their symptoms to a flu-like virus. However, their blood tests did not show the presence of any viral infection.

New theories about the cause of fibromyalgia are continually evolving. A recent theory is that patients with fibromyalgia have a decreased level of brain serotonin. Serotonin is a chemical in the brain known as a neurotransmitter. It assists communication from one nerve to another. Research has shown a decrease in serotonin is associated with symptoms common to fibromyalgia – musculoskeletal pain, sleep disturbances, and depression.

With few biological clues, many physicians assumed that fibromyalgia was a psychosomatic illness of depression and anxiety. New findings show that the majority of people with fibromyalgia do not experience abnormal levels of these moods. Many of the standardized tests used to measure depression among people with fibromyalgia were designed for the physically healthy population, not for people in pain. The pain of fibromyalgia creates a very different kind of fatigue, and subsequent depression, than that of being tired because of increased physical activity or insufficient sleep. Resting does not reduce the fatigue or the pain, and without drugs it is often difficult to induce a sound sleep.

Researchers are now looking at the "which-came-first" question: Do depression and anxiety bring on pain, or are they the result of pain? At a recent conference on fibromyalgia, the question was raised: "Is fibromyalgia a psychiatric disease?" The answer – based on research that is finally beginning to catch up with clinical observations – was a resounding "NO!" Even though some may feel depressed, the vast majority of fibromyalgia patients don't meet the criteria for depression. What's causing their kind of depression may simply be a feeling of loss of control over what is happening to their body, a lack of answers to the cause of the debilitating pain and fatigue, and a lack of understanding and compassion from friends, family, and the medical community.

A less popular theory is that fibromyalgia may be the result of an abnormal autoimmune mechanism. Patients may become hypersensitive to their own tissue, foods and/or chemicals which trigger reactions as if the body were responding to foreign invaders. With the exception of physicians with an interest in environmental health, this theory is summarily dismissed by the medical community.

### Symptoms

Even though most of the information I uncovered about fibromyalgia wasn't very encouraging, in a strange way I was reassured as I read further about this condition. Through the stuffy scientific language, I could feel a common bond with the people who were suffering the way I was. Nowhere was this feeling stronger than when I read about the symptoms.

### Pain

The major symptom of fibromyalgia is pain. Most people feel the pain of fibromyalgia as aching, stiffness, and tenderness around joints, muscles, tendons, and ligaments. Pain may appear in one location or in many different parts of the body. The pain may be located within the muscles themselves, as well as the points where ligaments attach muscles to bones.

Unless they are questioned about pain in other locations, their fibromyalgia may be overlooked, misdiagnosed, and mistreated, because most patients are likely to concentrate on the area that is causing the most pain at the time they are examined. Questions about pain in various locations of the body are important in a physical exam, since widespread pain raises the possibility of fibromyalgia. Most patients with fibromyalgia have axial skeletal pain (in the same position on both sides of the body off the spinal axis). If this is present, it can be another clue to help confirm the diagnosis.

Fibromyalgia patients describe their pain in a variety of ways: radiating, burning, shooting, stabbing, pressing, gnawing, tingling, or deep muscular pain. The pain may also feel worse at different times of the day, or strike different body parts as a result of different kinds of activity, i.e., the hands or arms when typing or driving; the back or shoulders when sitting at a desk for too long; the legs after periods of walking or biking. Pain and stiffness may be worse in the morning. For some people, the morning pain disappears in 10 to 15 minutes; for others it may last all day.

People with fibromyalgia feel extreme tenderness in many specific anatomical locations. These "tender points" are the major determining feature of fibromyalgia. The locations of tender points are similar in all persons with fibromyalgia and are an important part of the diagnosis. Multiple tender points are the characteristic physical finding in fibromyalgia; they do not occur in any other disorder.

For diagnostic purposes, fibromyalgia patients must have

pain in 11 of the 18 tender points that cluster around the neck, shoulder, chest, hip, knee, and elbow regions. This is the primary feature that distinguishes fibromyalgia from generalized rheumatism patients.

The importance of the examination for tender points has only recently been recognized. It has been demonstrated that the tenderness found in fibromyalgia patients is specific to the tender point sites and not merely a part of a generalized, all-over tenderness. Using dolorimeter methodology – a technique that applies heat to the skin and measures the intensity of pain perception in degrees ranging from unpleasant to unbearable – tests found that fibromyalgia patients had more pain over tender point sites, but not over neutral sites, when compared to non-fibromyalgia controls.

**Fatigue**

Fatigue can be the most debilitating aspect of fibromyalgia. Some people experience fatigue as a lack of muscle endurance while others describe the fatigue as an overall lack of energy. Much of the fatigue is attributed to a lack of restful, restorative sleep.

Sleep can be separated into two major stages: non-REM (non-rapid-eye-movement) sleep and REM (rapid-eye-movement) sleep. As a person starts the sleep cycle, or falls asleep, s/he will begin with a non-REM phase which lasts approximately 90 minutes. S/he will then progress into a REM sleep which lasts approximately 30 minutes. A person cycles in and out of non-REM and REM sleep throughout the night about four to six times, with the later REM periods lasting longer. The total amount of time spent in REM sleep should be about 25 percent. Any disruption of sleep cycles can lead to unwanted symptoms.

There are four stages of non-REM sleep which can be described from light to deep, and are referred to as Stages I to IV, or alpha to delta (from the Greek alphabet). Stage I, alpha, is the lightest level of sleep; Stage IV, or delta, is the deepest.

Slow-wave sleep (SWS) consists of Stages III and IV, and it is a deep, restful sleep. Growth hormone secretion is triggered by SWS, and its release from the pituitary gland is essential for tissue growth and cell repair. Other important hormone and immune system substances (such as antibodies) are also produced during non-REM sleep. This stage of sleep is needed for stimulating many restorative processes.

REM sleep is often referred to as the dreaming stage. The eyes may flash back and forth as though watching a movie projected onto your eyelids. Despite what appears to be intensive brain activity, most of the body's muscles enter a state of paralysis. While the body is still, the brain is active, almost to the point of being awake, but not quite.

Although not completely understood, it is believed that during REM sleep the brain reorganizes thoughts and events that took place during the preceding day. Memory and mood state may both be impacted by REM sleep.

Stage IV sleep is referred to as restorative sleep because it is during this sleep stage that the growth hormone needed for tissue growth and repair is released and chemicals needed by the immune system are produced. Both of these functions relate to fibromyalgia.

Tests of people with fibromyalgia often show a sleep disorder in which the deep and restful sleep of Stage IV is disturbed or interrupted. This disturbance is referred to as alpha (Stage I) intrusion of delta (Stage IV) sleep, or alpha-delta sleep. It is possible that the low energy levels experienced by people with fibromyalgia are the result of these sleep disturbances.

There is also evidence that continued sleep disturbances can lead to muscle pain. In one study, volunteers who did not have fibromyalgia were subjected to artificial disturbance of their Stage IV sleep. They developed pain and soreness in their muscles very similar to that felt by people with fibromyalgia. The result of this combination of pain and fatigue causes people with fibromyalgia to limit their physical activities, which turns into a vicious cycle of reduced endurance and increased symptoms.

Alpha-delta sleep is not specific to fibromyalgia, but it is seen in more than half of fibromyalgia patients. It is also sometimes seen in patients with psychiatric disorders, people experiencing emotional stress, and in patients with sleep apnea (interrupted breathing), rheumatoid arthritis, nocturnal myoclonus (jerking movements of arms and legs during sleep), and teeth grinding. This alpha-delta intrusion occurs in 60 percent of the sleep of fibromyalgia patients, in contrast to an alpha-delta intrusion rate of 25 percent in the sleep patterns of insomniacs, normal controls, and others.

People with an alpha-delta sleep disorder awaken feeling unrefreshed even after eight to ten hours in bed, almost as though they hadn't slept at all. They are tired and frequently have morning stiffness and pain.

In a study of 60 fibromyalgia patients who were asked, "When in the day do you feel best?" most patients said that their best time of day was around noon. This is a marked contrast to most healthy people, who often feel a lull around noontime – either because they are hungry and need the stimulus provided by elevating their blood glucose levels with food, or because they are feeling bloated and sleepy after having already eaten. (Lue 1993)

The exact role of sleep in creating or aggravating the symptoms of fibromyalgia is still not clear. Although most fibromyalgia patients do report a problem with sleep, their symptoms can vary from sleep fragmentation to alpha-wave intrusion into disturbed deep sleep. Some fibromyalgia patients don't appear to have alpha-wave intrusions and some healthy controls display this problem without having any painful, fatiguing symptoms.

**Mitral Valve Prolapse**

Another symptom, mitral valve prolapse, frequently appears with fibromyalgia. This valve keeps blood from backing up from the heart's left lower chamber (the left ventricle) into the left upper chamber (the left atrium).

Other possible symptoms of fibromyalgia are presented in Appendix D.

I had learned a great deal about what fibromyalgia is, and what might be its cause. Now I needed to know what to do about it. With my own personal experiences as a barometer, it was no surprise to discover that there are gaps in knowledge when it comes to treatment for this syndrome.

# Chapter 7
# SEARCHING FOR KNOWLEDGE: THE DIAGNOSIS DILEMMA

*Knowledge is of two kinds. We know a subject ourselves or we know where we can find information upon it.*
— SAMUEL JOHNSON, *BOSWELL, LIFE*, 1775

Reaching a diagnosis can indeed be a challenge.

There are no specific laboratory tests or imaging procedures (e.g. x-rays, CAT scan, magnetic resonance imaging) that can detect fibromyalgia. As I discovered from both my research and my personal experience, for many years it was thought that the disorder was psychological.

Numerous factors contribute to the skepticism of the examining physician (who may not be knowledgeable about fibromyalgia), and the doubt about whether this is a physical and real condition. They include: swelling reported in areas that seem unswollen to the examiner; common complaints of morning stiffness and fatigue; histrionic descriptive terms such as "tearing" or "exploding;" psychophysiological features such as anxiety, headache, and irritable bowel syndrome; and subtle problems with memory, concentration ability, and depression.

It has only been in recent years, since the mid- or late 1980s, as more has been learned about fibromyalgia, that the medical profession has begun to accept it as a physical disease or syndrome.

The first step to a diagnosis, as for any medical condition, is taking a careful history. The patient must be convinced that the physician has listened to, and believed, all that she/he has reported. A thorough physical examination must then follow. Tests may include:

- Blood, urine and stool analysis
- Antinuclear antibody screen
- Rheumatoid factor and thyroxin levels
- Electrocardiogram (EKG), chest x-ray, or other electro-diagnostic studies for patients who report chest pain or numbness and tingling
- Bone and joint x-rays, if the patient perceives significant joint swelling

For a patient whose primary condition is fibromyalgia, all of these tests will return normal, providing evidence for both the patient and the doctor that no underlying or associated disease, such as anemia, viral infection, thyroid disease, or other rheumatic disease has been overlooked.

Morning stiffness occurs in more than 80 percent of fibromyalgia patients. However, it may also occur in patients with back and neck problems, various osteoarthritic disorders, or rheumatoid arthritis. This morning stiffness, while helpful in the diagnosis of fibromyalgia in younger individuals, may complicate the diagnosis in the elderly.

In 1990, the American College of Rheumatology found

that two criteria, used in combination, were the best available for both classifying and diagnosing fibromyalgia:

1. A history of widespread pain that the patient has experienced for at least three months in all of the following areas of the body: the left and right sides of the body, including shoulder and buttock pain; the spine, which includes the upper neck area; the lower back below the waist; and the chest area.

2. Pain on examination by touch in 11 of the 18 tender point sites. Pressure must be with a four-kilogram force, 11 of the 18 areas must be positive, and the patient must state that the pressure was "painful," because "tender" is not sufficient.

One of the biggest problems in diagnosing fibromyalgia is distinguishing it from other diseases and conditions. One condition with symptoms similar to fibromyalgia is chronic fatigue syndrome (CFS). At one time, it was thought that the Epstein-Barré virus was the cause of chronic fatigue syndrome, but this theory has been recently discounted. Many experts have noted striking similarities between fibromyalgia and CFS; i.e., it strikes primarily females, and has a long-time duration of symptoms that include fatigue, pain, sleep disturbances, morning stiffness, irritable bowels, numbness and tingling, and tender points. However, CFS patients may also have a fever.

Dr. Steven Strauss, chief clinical investigator for the National Institute of Allergy and Infectious Disease (NIAID), recently spoke at a workshop on fibromyagia sponsored by the National Institutes of Health. He opened his speech with an anecdote that may best describe the controversy between fibromyalgia and CFS.

"While most of you [rheumatologists] have been tinkering with the left front axle and we [infectious disease specialists] have been tinkering with the right front axle, we are all too reluctant to look closer at what is under the hood!" (Straus 1993)

Dr. Strauss added, "The symptoms of CFS and fibromyalgia syndrome are broadly overlapping, and I think that the diagnosis depends largely on which physician the patient chooses to go to, based upon bias and what they perceive as bothering them the most." (Straus 1993)

The general muscle tightness that occurs in other parts of the body can also localize in the jaw muscles, which results in temporomandibular joint (TMJ) symptoms. There may be difficulty in opening the mouth wide, an inability to slide the lower jaw side to side, clicking noises when opening the jaw, and sometimes ringing in the ear.

TMJ may occasionally be the early signs of fibromyalgia, but treatments that alleviate the pain of TMJ (for example, appliances placed in the mouth to prevent grinding of the teeth or jaw tension while sleeping) do not help the fibromyalgia condition. If neck and shoulder pain is also present, a more comprehensive check for fibromyalgia is in order.

Pain and numbness in the index and middle fingers along with weakness in the thumb could be symptoms of carpal tunnel syndrome and may result in surgery. True carpal tunnel patients usually show significant improvement after this surgery, but fibromyalgia patients do not. Carpal tunnel diagnosis should be followed up with clear-cut testing to identify this syndrome and conclusively rule out fibromyalgia.

Fibromyalgia is often misdiagnosed as Lyme disease. Two studies showed that many people seeking treatment for, and being diagnosed as having, Lyme disease actually had fibromyalgia.

One study of 92 patients seeking treatment for Lyme disease at Rush Lyme Center in Chicago found only six confirmed cases of the disease. Thirty-five of the patients in the study were found to have fibromyalgia.

In a related study, Dr. Leonard Sigal, a rheumatologist at the Robert Wood Johnson Medical School in New Brunswick, NJ, noted that more than 10 percent of the people who had been tested for Lyme disease at the school's Lyme disease center actually had fibromyalgia. (1993)

A missed diagnosis of fibromyalgia leads to unnecessary antibiotic therapy for presumed Lyme arthritis or neurologic disease, and delays a diagnosis and appropriate therapy for fibromyalgia.

On the other hand, the discomfort felt during Lyme disease may interfere with sleep sufficiently to precipitate fibromyalgia, or fibromyalgia may already be present during Lyme disease, with the similar viral-like symptoms of musculoskeletal pain and fatigue.

Patients with fibromyalgia frequently report problems associated with cold: worsening symptoms in cold weather, having cold hands, and generally feeling colder than other people. Some patients with fibromyalgia have an elaborate, netlike discoloration of the skin which may be an exaggerated reaction of blood vessels to cold. Questionnaire-based studies of patients with fibromyalgia have demonstrated a 30 to 50 percent prevalence of symptoms similar to Reynaud's Syndrome, a disorder noted by constricted arteries.

Reynaud's, too, could be a misdiagnosis. In fibromyalgia patients, however, these Reynaud's Syndrome-like symptoms – pain or discomfort during exposure to cold – quickly disappear with warming.

The wide array of symptoms associated with fibromyalgia is frequently misdiagnosed as other individual syndromes, again making a fibromyalgia diagnosis more difficult. Fibromyalgia is overlooked, and patients are treated for other, nonexistent, syndromes.

When the medical system fails to find clinically positive proof (laboratory tests and x-rays) for the existence of fibromyalgia, and the physicians are not knowledgeable about the tender-point check, many patients are told they are suffering from depression. "It's all in your head. This is all related to stress." How many times have we heard this, or known that someone, a doctor or a family member, thought it?

Two different groups of patients with fibromyalgia who were studied in 1985 and 1992 had a greater family history of major depression, but the vast majority of these people were not themselves diagnosed as clinically depressed. There have been a large number of studies on psychological and psychiatric aspects of fibromyalgia, finding that the majority of patients do not have any current psychiatric illness. Nevertheless, a certain number of patients, estimated at about 30 percent, are in fact depressed.

Even if the majority of fibromyalgia patients aren't clinically depressed, there is a link. They have a greater personal lifetime history and family history of depression. (This is also true with other pain disorders like rheumatoid arthritis.) too.) It is difficult to determine if depression is chemically linked to fibromyalgia, or if this is a reactive response to chronic pain and fatigue. Reactive depression and anxiety are not surprising in a disorder that causes constant pain, is inadequately treated, and is so poorly understood.

No relationship has been established between fibromyalgia and other rheumatic diseases such as rheumatoid arthritis, osteoarthritis, ankylosing spondylitis, polymyalgia, and systemic lupus erythematosus. Blood tests, such as the ANA (antinuclear antibodies) test, generally rule out these other diseases. Yet, it is not uncommon for these disorders to occur together with fibromyalgia. Given the wide variety of symptoms, the frustration of finding a physician who can diagnose this "mystery disease," and the lack of empathy from family, friends, and the medical community, it is no accident that anxiety and depression are part and parcel of the syndrome.

## Chapter 8
## SEARCHING FOR KNOWLEDGE: THE TREATMENT DILEMMA

*It is the peculiarity of knowledge that those who really thirst for it always get it.*
— RICHARD JEFFRIES, *COUNTRY LITERATURE*

The medical community generally agrees that there is no cure for fibromyalgia – no magic bullet that will make the symptoms disappear forever. A number of treatments, however, are currently being used. To date, these treatments can best be described as methods to cope with the symptoms. The coping methods include medications, exercise, and various other therapies.

### MEDICATIONS

Because of the common occurrence of the alpha-delta sleep anomaly in fibromyalgia, a fair amount of research has focused on the use of trycyclic anti-depressants such as amitriptyline (Elavil) and cyclobenzaprine (Flexeril) for fibromyalgia patients. These two medications, which have similar chemical characteristics, are used in doses so small that they are not effective as anti-depressants, but are thought to help some patients sleep better.

As far back as 1986, a study reported in the professional journal *Arthritis and Rheumatism* found that 50 milligrams of amitriptyline at bedtime helped with the fatigue, pain, and general lack of feelings of well-being in patients with fibromyalgia, but did not reduce the pain of tender points.

The study did not test the effects of amytriptyline beyond six weeks of use, and the drug is known to have annoying long-term side effects for some, including dry mouth, constipation and weight gain. (Goldenberg, Felson, and Dinerman 1986)

Donald Goldenberg, M.D., a rheumatologist from Tufts University Medical School in Boston, is one of the nation's leading researchers and clinicians in fibromyalgia. He spoke on this subject in June 1991 – when I was deeply involved with my search for relief from my symptoms. He addressed a public forum, "Fibromyalgia and Chronic Fatigue Syndrome," at Columbia Hospital in Milwaukee. I could not attend his lecture, but purchased his tape and had it transcribed. He noted that the low dose of amitriptyline used in treating fibromyalgia releases serotonin at levels that might be sufficient to relax muscles and enable restorative sleep. Research indicated that it is moderately effective in about 50 percent of fibromyalgia patients. It may have a direct relaxation effect on muscles, as well as an independent anti-inflammatory effect. He emphasized that this is not a cure. The medication may allow deeper and more refreshing sleep for most people, and some pain relief in others.

According to an article in *Arthritis Today*, many people with fibromyalgia complain that medications provide little relief from their painful symptoms. For some fibromyalgia patients, treatment with the most commonly used medications may be no more helpful than no treatment at all.

Short-term clinical trials have shown that two drugs – the anitdepressant amitriptyline and the muscle relaxant cyclobenzaprine – are sometimes helpful in relieving fibromyalgia symptoms in a small percentage of patients.

Doctors at 11 Canadian medical centers compared the effects of the two medications in 208 patients. The patients were divided into three groups; one group received amitriptyline, another received cyclobenzaprine and the third received a placebo.

Prior to this six-month study, and at monthly intervals throughout the study, participants were rated on such factors as pain, fatigue, sleeping difficulty, morning stiffness, and psychological status. Ratings were based on examinations by physicians, as well as by the patients' own reports.

After the first month of treatment, 21 percent of the amitriptyline-treated patients, 12 percent of the cyclobenzaprine-treated patients and none of the patients receiving a placebo showed measurable improvement. The most significant findings came at the third and sixth months of the study: improvement had increased in all three groups and was almost evenly matched.

"I would have to say, in scientific controlled studies right now, these are the best medicines that anybody has used," Dr. Goldenberg concluded. "And they aren't great. You can bet that people are looking for better medications, but as far as I'm concerned, right now there's nothing – no breakthrough, major, or exciting, regarding medication available..."

He did add a note of cautious hope. "There are a lot of

interesting studies going on throughout the world. One other interesting study demonstrated, actually, that cardiovascular fitness exercise achieves just about as good results in fibromyalgia as do these medications." (Goldenberg 1992)

Medications other than amitriptyline, such as nonsteroidal anti-inflammatory drugs (NSAIDs) like ibuprofen and naproxen, have been shown to be of little benefit in the treatment of fibromyalgia. In one controlled study, Goldenberg found no benefits from naproxen when compared with a placebo. In fact, the lack of response to a long list of NSAIDs is often a diagnostic tip-off for the patient with long-standing fibromyalgia.

If other forms of arthritis that might respond to NSAIDs are also present, the physician must be certain which symptoms are being treated.

Narcotics are not appropriate for treatment of fibromyalgia. Many fibromyalgia patients find the acute pains of tooth extraction or surgery more tolerable than the chronic pain of their disease and believe that the only drug that will give them relief is a narcotic. But fibromyalgia researcher and UCLA professor Stuart L. Silverman, M.D., has found that the pain of fibromyalgia usually does not respond to narcotics. In his studies, he found that only 15 percent of fibromyalgia patients felt that narcotics significantly reduced their pain, and only 25 percent felt the pain medicine significantly improved the quality of their lives.

Before the diagnosis criteria for fibromyalgia was established, many patients went through multiple evaluations, as I did, for the same complaints with varying results. If the symptoms arose after an injury, or if litigation or disability was an issue, patients were suspected of malingering or exaggerating the symptoms.

If they were treated at all, it was often inappropriately. They may have been told they had arthritis and treated with systemic corticosteroids or gold injections. If chest wall pain was a prominent symptom, they may have had cardiac catherization, an invasive and sometimes risky procedure to determine if there is blockage of the coronary arteries. Persistent neck or back pain sometimes resulted in one or more unsuccessful attempts at surgical intervention.

The use of NSAIDs, physical therapy, muscle relaxants, and pain killers, even if they helped at first, were generally ineffective.

**EXERCISE**

Poor posture and lack of physical fitness are common traits of fibromyalgia patients, so to strive for a higher level of aerobic fitness is essential.

Many patients with fibromyalgia, however, are reluctant to exercise because of the initial sensation of more pain.

Although I had started exercise walking six years before the onset of fibromyalgia symptoms in 1984, and had started swimming laps six years before that, since 1984 each time I started to exercise, my body ached all over. The first 10 to 15 minutes of walking or five laps of swimming were painful. However, the longer I walked or swam the more the pain diminished.

The combination of pain and fatigue in fibromyalgia can become a "Catch-22." Lack of appropriate exercise leads to stasis or slow-down in the lymph system, which may produce more tired feelings and a lack of desire to exercise.

Deep breathing and gentle stretching exercises, plus

rebounder and/or walking activities are appropriate for almost everybody. Walking, swimming, or stationary bicycling will increase aerobic fitness. One can gradually increase time and/or distance as physical condition improves. Strenuous activity every day is not recommended.

Chapter 17 presents a complete discussion of exercise choices.

## OTHER REMEDIES

Although there have been no controlled studies, the following therapies have been helpful for *some* people with fibromyalgia *some* of the time:

**Acupuncture** – A traditional Chinese therapeutic technique where the body is punctured with very fine needles that cause no pain. It may be very helpful for relieving pain at the tender or trigger points.

**Biofeedback** – Requires an experienced therapist and the use of an electronic machine, and may help someone to consciously control the relaxation of muscles and to increase blood flow through the body.

**Epsom-salt and baking-soda baths** – A daily bath of ½ cup each of Epsom salt and baking soda in a tub of warm (not hot) water for 10 to 15 minutes.

**Heat treatments** – Hot packs and showers may give some short-term relief.

**Homeopathy** – A holistic approach to healing that emphasizes the interrelatedness of mind and body and all the body systems. Homeopathy uses small quantities of natural medicines to stimulate the body's own healing powers.

**"Joints and Glands Exercises"** – An audio tape with a supporting book that has proved tremendously helpful to me in sustaining my recovery. The book and tape are available through The Himalayan Institute, 800-822-4547.

**Mental health therapies** – These may include psychotherapy or stress therapy, or fibromyalgia support groups.

**Physical therapies** – The best of these realign the body toward improved posture or myofascial release. This passively stretches the stiff and tight muscles and relaxes them.

**Rest** – Can be combined with meditation, visualization, and/or relaxation techniques.

**Serotonin** – Dr. Neal Barnard, in his 1998 book, *Foods That Fight Pain,* has some helpful and interesting information about serotonin.

> Many fibromyalgia symptoms could be explained by a lack of serotonin, a brain chemical that suppresses pain. Serotonin is also essential for regulating moods (which could explain why depression hits about 40 percent of people with fibromyalgia) and plays a role in sleep, which is also often disturbed in fibromyalgia.
>
> ...foods can boost serotonin naturally. Foods that are high in carbohydrates – breads, pasta, potatoes or fruits – can increase the serotonin in the brain. High carbohydrate foods also increase a second brain chemical called norepinephrine, which is also important in pain control and in moods.

**Topical treatments** – These include spraying tender points with ethyl chloride, or applying creams sold under the names of AURUM, EMLA, and PAIN-FREE, all of which need to be used in repeated doses on a daily basis, and only on limited areas of the body at one time. One major advantage of topical treatments is that they do not cause stomach or gastrointestinal irritation.

In many of the articles I've read, education was emphasized as an important ingredient in the search for wellness. Dr. Goldenberg says, "Education consists of a complete and realistic discussion of the diagnosis and prognosis. The patient should be reassured that fibromyalgia is neither life-threatening nor degenerative, and no structural or cosmetic abnormalities will develop over time."

At the end of all of this reading, researching, summarizing, and analyzing, I knew much more than I'd known before. Unfortunately, I was no closer to a solution.

# Part III

## GETTING ON WITH LIFE

## Chapter 9
## 1991: HOPE ON THE HORIZON

*Ere now I would have ended my miseries in death,*
*but found Hope keeps the spark alive,*
*whispering ever that tomorrow will be better than today.*
— TIBULLUS, *ELEGIES*. BK II, ELEG. 6, L. 19

The two phone calls I made that significant morning in 1991 led to two consultations.

Frank Fantazzi, the physical therapist, was able to see me within a few days. He took notes as I shared my physical history with him. The picture painted by these notes describes where I was at that moment in time, and the searching I had done to get there.

> Ms. Musickant is a 58-year-old self-employed female who has a five- to six-year history of chronic pain. She reports that she has lower-back pain, middle-back pain, neck pain, facial pain and headaches.
> 
> She has been treated by many physicians including several internists, chiropractors and an orthopedist.
> 
> She has been treated by Dr. Sweeney for approximately

the last two years, with marked improvement in her overall condition reported since she has been seeing Dr. Sweeney for symptoms of fibromyalgia.

Ms. Musickant states that she swims a couple of times a week and she does an excessive amount of stretching exercises, which do help her feel better. She states, however, that the amount of time that she spends exercising and stretching interferes with her real living. Her goal for treatment here is to reduce the amount of time that she does spend so that she can return to real living.

Ms. Musickant reports the pain began approximately six years ago in the right hip and the right foot. This led to low back pain and eventually middle back and neck pain and headaches.

There has been a gradual progression of pain since initial onset. She reports that the pain is intermittent in nature. It is especially worse with sitting. She feels best with exercise and walking approximately one-half hour a day. Today she reports her pain is a 4 on a 0 to 10 scale. She states that it ranges between a 1 and a 5 most of the time. She states that this intermittent pain is fairly constant.

Diagnostic Tests: Ms. Musickant reports that she has had blood tests and x-rays, all of which have been negative.

Medications: Presently patient reports taking Premarin, Provera, and Anacin.

Past Medical History: Is significant in that she has irritable bowel, food sensitivities, and allergies most notable over the past eight years. She also reports a history of a fractured arm at age two and a fractured coccyx [tail bone] approximately thirty years ago. Other than this, no other significant history.

He then studied my standing posture, head and neck movements bending forward, backward, and to the side. He checked my lower back to determine my range of motion and to identify any discomfort I was experiencing. He examined the motion of my jaw (temporomandibular joint).

He concluded what I already knew – much about me wasn't working quite as it should. In his words:

> Dysfunction at all levels of the cervical, [neck] thoracic, [chest] and lumbar spine including the pelvic girdle [lower back].

His treatment plan:

> First treat the pelvic girdle and the sacroiliac [lower back] area with muscle energy techniques and joint mobilization of the lumbar spine [the part of the back between the lowest ribs and the pelvis]. Stretching of the right hip muscles also indicated to completely balance pelvis.
>
> Also treat spine of the neck and chest area and the left jaw. These areas, too, show restricted motion.
>
> This should be followed up by mobilization and stretching of the thoracic spine with most likely treatment at the cervical-thoracic junction.

He planned to see me twice a week for the next two to

three weeks.

Seven treatments later, much of my pain was relieved and the pain relief held. The muscles relaxed, the headaches were less frequent and the TMJ pain never returned.

It sounds so simple in retrospect, but the process of treating jaw and chest, neck and torso, shoulders and hips, was not without discomfort. The pain of stretching the muscle inside my left jaw was so excruciating it brought tears to my eyes. Imagine a rubber band stretched tautly and held for a period of time until, when it is released, it does not snap back completely to its original state.

But, painful as the process was, it left no residual discomfort. The physical therapy was exactly what I needed at this point.

The other half of the solution came at this time as well. I waited a month to see Dr. Norman Schwartz, and he said he was squeezing me in to see me that soon. Dr. Schwartz is a graduate of the University of Pennsylvania School of Medicine and has a family medicine practice in Milwaukee. His treatment method focuses on nutritional therapy. Observing the progress – or lack of progress – of some of his patients, opened his mind to some humbling new insights.

"What we don't know is greater than what we do know," he said. "The more we learn, the more questions there are that remain unanswered." (1996)

Dr. Schwartz believes that the idea of a medical difference between the mind and the body is an anachronistic one. They are one and the same, he says. When he talked about "chronic unwellness" and "the walking wounded" I felt he was describing the past seven years of my life.

He had become intrigued with the role of nutrition and

environment in health after a 1990 meeting of the American Academy of Environmental Health. He found he wasn't the only doctor dealing with chronic unwellness. More and more physicians were looking to diet and environmental toxins as possible causes of, or contributors to, ill health. This was the framework, the belief system, he was looking for. It was a marked shift from the pharmaceutical emphasis of medical school, where drugs were seen as magic bullets to combat disease.

Dr. Schwartz says we have squandered our health by exposing ourselves to chemical additives and toxins in the food we eat and the air we breathe – from the fertilizers that promote crop growth, to the chemicals that fatten livestock, to the pollutants belched into the air by the vehicles we drive.

He says we are ingesting all of these substances through our digestive and respiratory systems, and it would be a miracle if there were NOT adverse effects.

Another idea that Dr. Schwartz emphasizes is the variability of every human being. Some people, many people, are impervious to all these assaults to their systems and go through life feeling just fine. Others are more sensitive, and the various exposures that they experience affect their immune systems more, and result in a variety of symptoms and ailments. I seemed to fall into this latter group.

I saw Dr. Schwartz in early September of 1991. What he said made sense to me. After he read my responses to an extensive health appraisal questionnaire (which he had mailed to me in advance of my appointment), he recommended that I have a blood test called the ELISA/ACT™ (Enzyme-Linked Immunosorbant Assay/Activated Cell Test). This test and the questionnaire were developed by laboratory pathologist

Russell Jaffe at the Serammune Physicians Lab, which he founded in Virginia in 1984. I would later learn more about this medical genius, whose revolutionary ideas were transforming peoples' lives and could have the potential to change the face of medicine itself.

A research scientist at the National Institutes of Health from 1973 to 1979, Dr. Jaffe was a boy wonder who once had the distinction of being the youngest permanent member of the National Institutes of Health senior staff.

Now his interests are with the mechanisms of health, rather than exclusively with the mechanisms of disease. Dr. Jaffe focuses on ways to enhance the immune system.

According to Dr. Jaffe, the immune system is constantly learning about our environment. The immune function can then be defined as knowing and maintaining the distinction between us and the outside world. The needs of defense, repair, and communication are the responsibility of the immune system.

If we can tolerate the environment, we are healthy. In this state of health we tolerate ourselves and our surroundings, and our immune system repairs us and neutralizes foreign invaders. Healthy people have robust, resilient, active cellular systems that clean up internal debris from the wear and tear of the body, as well as anything our immune system identifies as "not self."

If we are sensitive (the medical usage of the term) to the environment, we have "allergies." People who are sensitive may have watery eyes, or sneezing, or a runny nose. They may have an infection that requires medical attention or an allergy that is unresponsive to treatment. Hypersensitivity, a higher degree of sensitivity, is called "autoimmunity." The hyper sensitive individual may have symptoms as diverse as migraine headaches, multiple sclerosis, irritable bowel syndrome (IBS), or chronic fatigue syndrome (CFS), among others.

Sensitive and hypersensitive people have four basic types of allergic responses:

Type I, "acute," occurs immediately following exposure to allergens. The reactions may be sneezing, itching, hives, or even life-threatening swelling following a bee sting.

Type II, "delayed reaction," may take hours or days to develop. Some examples are Rh blood factor incompatibility reactions, drug-induced reactions, and many autoimmune conditions.

Type III, also "delayed reaction," may take hours or days to develop. Rheumatoid arthritis and rheumatic fever are examples of this type of reaction.

Type IV reaction is mediated by T cells that have been previously sensitized to the specific antigen. In other words, the T-cells come to do battle against the allergen. This type of reaction is seen in a TB skin test, contact dermatitis, and tissue or organ-rejection reactions. It is the classic "delayed reaction" that can take days to develop.

As I talked with Dr. Schwartz and researched further into the field of immunology, I was learning more and more about this amazing system. Our immune defense and repair system is constantly challenged by substances in the environment, such as food and chemicals. If this defense and repair function is overwhelmed, we become more susceptible to infectious disease, allergic reactions, or hypersensitivity.

Immune overload can result in recurrent infections or multisystem chronic inflammatory and/or autoimmune syndromes like fibromyalgia.

Dr. Marshall Mandell and Lynne Waller Scanlon, in their book, *Dr. Mandell's 5-Day Allergy Relief System* (1978), answer some interesting questions:

> Why should a person be allergic to anything he eats, drinks, or inhales? After all, everything with which he comes into contact is derived in some form from something that is part of our Earth. The answers, we have discovered, involve mankind's increasing inability to cope with natural as well as unnatural substances in his environment.
>
> How did this happen? For hundreds of thousands of years during the course of human evolution, changes occurred much more slowly in man's natural environment than they do in the rapidly changing chemicalized and polluted world of today. If a volcano erupted, filling the air with flames, gases, and particles, and pouring forth rivers of lava, those contaminants entered the Earth's atmosphere and water, and covered some areas of land, but the Earth, still young and fresh, was able to accommodate what were, in the grand scheme of things, minor changes. The relatively limitless atmosphere, huge land masses, and enormous bodies of water easily absorbed and diluted or distributed the naturally formed volcanic pollutants. Man had sufficient time to adjust to the pollution that resulted from the activity of a natural occurrence on his planet such as a volcanic eruption. He slowly evolved over a period of hundreds of thousands of years. He adapted. He survived. When death came, it was from old age,

injury, tribal war, infection, in the jaws of a sabertoothed tiger, or the cooking pot of a neighbor. When disease struck, it usually was not black lung, cancer, or coronary heart disease – these are the diseases of our advanced civilization.

During the past two centuries alone, man has brought about such drastic changes in his natural environment that it has become unnatural. When organic chemistry began in the nineteenth century, a whole series of combinations of chemicals were created that were never found naturally in the environment. Pesticides, herbicides (weed killers), insecticides, waxes, preservatives, colorings, and additives, although they did the jobs they were designed for, contaminated the environment and filled man's body with residues that were totally alien to the human system. When jet fuels were developed for commercial aviation in the 1950's, combustion by-products began to be spewed across the land – by-products with no equal in the natural form. Automobiles manufactured by the millions each year compounded the problem. Oil and coal-burning factories and generating plants added to this. In short, everything man eats, drinks, or inhales is now polluted with chemical agents that are foreign to his chemistry, and he is suffering the consequences of possessing a body that is incapable of handling the by-products of his amazing chemical technology.

But that is just part of the story. The second part concerns a lowered threshold of allergic resistance to physical and mental illness, and an inability to cope with the natural, as well as the unnatural things that surround him because of an out-of-kilter body metabolism, enzyme dysfunctions, nutritional deficiencies, and hormonal imbalances.

Where does that leave us? We are in a precarious position at best. Man no longer has the hundreds of thousands of years his body must have to adjust gradually to changes in the environment; there have been too many changes in the quality of the air, food, and water on which he depends. Compounding matters, his diet has changed radically over the past few generations and now includes so many heat and chemically modified and nutritionally inadequate foods from poor soil, that he is malnourished. In addition, in a weakened state, he has to deal with so many unnatural and toxic substances that his body is continually stressed. With few reserves to call on because of an inadequately nourished body, serious malfunctions often precipitate a maladapted state of hypersensitivity or allergy to many of the synthetic, as well as the natural substances in his environment. (Mandell and Scanlon 1978)

There is a way, which has been available for at least the past 10 years, to test individuals for substances to which they are sensitive. The ELISA/ACT™ blood test.

This test creates an immunologic fingerprint of an individual by testing white blood cells (lymphocytes) for their reactions to almost 400 purified foods, preservatives, chemicals, and minerals. The categories tested include: toxic minerals, environmental chemicals, additives and preservatives, dairy products, fish, crustaceans, mollusks, fowl, fruits, grains, meats, oils, nuts and seeds, pesticides, spices and seasonings, sugars, vegetables, and therapeutic foods.

On September 6, 1991, Dr. Schwartz drew my blood for the ELISA/ACT™ test and took a stool sample to determine the cause of my irritable bowel syndrome.

Nothing significant was revealed in the stool culture.

But the ELISA/ACT™ revealed a host of sensitivities.

Each food and chemical that creates a reaction of over 20 percent in the blood cells tested is considered a strong reaction; 5 to 20 percent is considered an intermediate reaction; less than 5 percent is not significant.

My highest scores showed up in the additives and preservatives category. Food coloring, monosodium glutamate (MSG), sodium benzoate, and sulfites were the worst offenders. Even then I knew enough about the food industry in this country to understand that these substances were widespread. In my research since, I have learned they are even more prevalent than I ever suspected.

I also showed strong reactions to cranberries, oysters, hops, allspice/arrowroot, garlic, and organophosphate (a pesticide).

My intermediate reactions included perch/mackerel, deer/venison, herbal teas, beets, cherries, coffee, brazil nuts, broccoli, mango, cola, caraway seeds, white potatoes, cantaloupe/honeydew, tapioca, and vanilla.

Of the 235 substances I was tested for at that time, I exhibited strong or intermediate reactions to 24 as well as to the entire category of additives and preservatives.

What an eye-opener! Why hadn't someone done this for me years ago? I wondered.

But armed with this information at last, I had to figure out how to use it. I had to see if eliminating these foods and chemicals would improve my health. Somehow I sensed I was on the right track. I felt perhaps now I had the knowledge to control what was controlling me. Would I be able to do it? Would it work?

I was determined to give this my best efforts. Still, the real test was yet to come. Two weeks later, with the ELISA/ACT™ results in hand, Joseph and I embarked on a vacation to England and Scotland.

## Chapter 10
## 1991: This Is A Remedy?

*When desperate ills demand a speedy cure,*
*Distrust is cowardice and prudence folly.*
— SAMUEL JOHNSON, *IRENE*. ACT IV, SC. 1, L. 87

Joseph and I love to travel together. Besides our annual trips to Florida, we have been to Spain, the Canary Islands, Russia, the Orient, Alaska, Israel, the Greek Isles, and Southeast Asia. We are always thinking about what part of the world we want to explore next, and where we might want to revisit. Even with my pain and discomfort, taking trips and planning for them is an important part of my life.

When I received the results of the ELISA/ACT™ test in 1991, we were getting ready to leave for three weeks in Great Britain. I felt certain that the ELISA/ACT™ results had the potential to turn this disease around for me in a way that nothing else had. But obviously it was going to require an all-out effort on my part. If I could do it, maybe I'd feel better on this vacation than I had for years. But what a challenge it would be!

In 1981, when I met Joseph, I was moving ahead in my

life with a certainty and competence that had been growing since I divorced my first husband. I was focused on educational and career goals for myself, which I had postponed for more than 25 years. On December 19, 1981 (my 49th birthday) I was awarded my B.A. degree. Along with the course work, I learned I was an effective communicator, both verbal and written. During high school I believed I couldn't write, but college was a challenge that forced me to overcome this mental block to produce the requisite papers. While attending college, I also taught assertiveness and transactional analysis (TA) in a women's development center. When I graduated, I was hired to develop a career program for displaced homemakers.

Joseph has dimples and smiles a lot. He can almost always make me laugh. There was a wonderful chemistry between us from the start, and the years since we married have proven to me – in a way that my first marriage never did – that two people sharing a life can give each other joy, contentment, and treasured companionship. Through the years of pain and frustration as I battled my mysterious disease, and through my almost obsessive campaign to learn all I could about it, Joseph has been my steadfast ally. He is always supportive and sympathetic, gently encouraging me when life seemed most distressing.

We headed for England and Scotland in September, and I tried to digest (no pun intended) what impact this list of food and chemical sensitivities the ELISA/ACT™ had uncovered would have on my life. Twenty-four items, plus the entire category of additives and preservatives, were targeted.

On the tour I eliminated or substituted for as many of the foods as I could identify, while still enjoying eating. I drank wonderful English Black teas instead of coffee, eliminated cantaloupe, honeydew, broccoli, and white potatoes, and avoided desserts (most of the time).

Sometimes, though, I would panic when I saw what was being served. Bus tours are notorious for running behind schedule. One stop too many, waiting an extra 10 minutes here and there for the stragglers, would make us late for meals. Ravenously hungry – always more so when I'm trying to watch what I'm eating – I would stare in disbelief when everything on the salad or appetizer plate was food I shouldn't eat.

Even though some of these were foods I enjoyed eating, I wasn't tempted. I was terrified of consuming anything the ELISA/ACT™ had identified as a problem for me. I so desperately wanted to stop hurting, to feel healthy and vital again. The pain of fibromyalgia kept me motivated to adhere to the discipline of this diet, not in the quantity of food, but in the choices. I created a mantra and would chant it silently in my head: "Do you want to feel good, or do you want to eat this?" Or I'd say to myself: "Don't poison yourself. Would you put arsenic in your mouth?"

Even the modest changes in diet I achieved while vacationing created unexpected results. When I stopped eating white potatoes, I no longer felt depressed. I originally thought the lack of depression was merely the result of the vacation in general – relaxation, many exciting diversions, and some of the most beautiful scenery I have ever experienced at the lochs and moors of Scotland. Several times since then, I have tried unadorned baked white potatoes only to find, each time, my depression returning.

We spent several days in London before and after the tour.

London is a wonderful city in which to stroll, saunter, trek, and trudge. We walked through art and history museums, the parks, the palaces, and the theater district. Taking the Tube, the London subway system, required much travel on foot to make connections from one line to another. Seven pounds (I don't mean English money) melted away, and my body felt trimmer. I was still taking acetaminophen for pain at night and doing stretching exercises before leaving the hotel each day, but the discomfort was much more manageable. I also felt less fatigued, in spite of the pace of the tour and the increased physical activity.

---

When we returned to Wisconsin, I was ready to focus my energies on recovery. I had a lengthy consultation with Dr. Schwartz about his recommendations for furthering the healing process. Besides eliminating as many of the items as I could that the ELISA/ACT™ had identified as troublesome to my immune system, Dr. Schwartz thought I should be supplementing my diet with vitamins, flavonoids, essential fatty acids, and other substances that would aid my digestion and the overall functioning of my body's systems.

But the specific suggestions made my head reel. The two-page "Supplement and Nutrition Recommendations" he gave me listed 15 different products, in very tiny print, with a different dosage and regimen and cautionary or explanatory comment for each one. Here are just some of the recommendations:

- Perque 1 (a blend of calcium, Magnesium, amino acids, lipotropics, and cofactors) – two tablets daily, 30 to 60 minutes before meals.

- Perque 2 (a blend of vitamins, minerals, and cofactors) – one or two tablets daily, with meal of choice.
- Active freeze-dried bacilli (lactobacillus-acidophilus) – two capsules before all meals for one month; two capsules before breakfast and dinner for two months.
- Coenzyme-10 – 60 milligrams before breakfast, lunch, and dinner.
- OmegaSyn-2 – one capsule with breakfast and dinner.
- L-Carnitine – one capsule one-half hour before breakfast and dinner.
- L-methionine – 500 milligrams upon rising and at bedtime.
- Hypericum/lomatium extract (an immune booster) – 20 drops in water, juice, or tea on Saturday and Sunday morning only. (Serammune Physician's Lab 1991)

Considering that fibromyalgia patients are subject to frequent mental confusion and have trouble thinking, it was no surprise this printout sent me into overload. I thought of my typical workday schedule (seven hours in front of a classroom of adults), and I could not fathom how I was going to not only take these supplements, but also try to keep track of them. Barely able to keep my anger under control, I looked at Dr. Schwartz, and maybe not as quietly and carefully as I might have, I asked him to reduce this list of 15 items to something more manageable. (He has since forgiven me for my testy disposition and behavior.)

He pared down the list to six items, taken to coincide with meals, shortly before eating, or with food. Dr. Schwartz also gave me some suggestions for organizing the supplements – using ice-cube trays or a divided "keep" box to distribute them for a week at a time.

The next shocker he presented to me was a diet plan. Dr. Schwartz recommended that I follow guidelines from William Crook's book, *The Yeast Connection.* Dr. Crook is a well-known physician and nutritional therapist who suggests that yeast intolerance is the culprit in a range of medical conditions from attention deficit disorder to ear infections. My first impression, as I stared in horror at this new assault on my fragile psyche, was that there was almost nothing I could eat if I followed his regimen and also removed from my diet the items identified by my ELISA/ACT™ test results.

- No sugar and sugar-containing foods
- No quick-acting carbohydrates which included sucrose, fructose, maltose, lactose, glycogen, glucose, mannitol, sorbitol, galactose, monosaccharides, and polysaccharides.
- No honey, molasses, maple syrup, maple sugar, date sugar, and turbinado sugar.
- No breads, biscuits, or muffins that contain yeast.
- No packaged or processed foods because canned, bottled, boxed, and other packaged and processed foods usually contain refined sugar products and other hidden ingredients.
- No cheeses or prepared foods that contain buttermilk, sour cream, or sour milk products, especially moldy cheeses, such as Roquefort, which are the worst.
- No alcoholic beverages or malt products such as cereal and candy.

- No processed or smoked meats such as sausage, hot dogs or pickled tongue.
- No edible fungi such as mushrooms, truffles, and morels.
- No coffee or tea, including herbal teas.
- No canned, bottled or frozen juice.
- No candied or dried fruits.

Seven years after the onset of the insidiously increasing pain, fatigue, anxiety, depression, and other mysterious symptoms, I was presented with this overwhelming challenge. It brought me close to tears.

Maybe the mantra from England would help. *Do you want to feel good, or do you want to eat this?* I felt the flavor was being stripped from my life. *Don't poison yourself. Would you put arsenic in your mouth?*

Could I really adhere to this program? Dr. Schwartz told me to stay on this rigid diet and supplement regimen until I returned from Florida in the spring. Four months! For someone whose social life revolved around eating, I was dumbfounded.

Would I be able to do it? I asked myself again. Dr. Schwartz was quietly encouraging, telling me about yeast-free breads and wonderful nut butters, such as cashew and almond, available at a local health food co-op. I knew a positive attitude would take me a long way, and I resolved to make use of my full resources and flagging energy the best I could.

With diet, nutritional supplements, and information in hand – and a great desire to give this my best shot – my husband and I set forth on our winter break.

## Chapter 11
## 1991: LEARNING ABOUT SULFITES AND OTHER HAZARDS TO MY HEALTH

*Prevention is so much better than healing.*
— THOMAS ADAMS, *WORKS*, P. 598 (1630)

There were two big reasons I was determined to give these diet modifications every chance I could. First, I was feeling slightly better after removing some of the foods in my diet to which I was sensitive. It wasn't anything dramatic or definitive, but it was enough to make me cautiously optimistic. Second, it was so important that this diet work for me because, at this point, I could see no other options for improving my health.

While I was setting up house again in Florida, I felt fearful of everything I ate. I constantly referred to my sulfited foods list, my Candida control diet (Dr. Crook's diet), and the ELISA/ACT™ results list. (Eventually the lists did become more familiar, and I didn't have to carry them with me all the time.)

I found that changing my eating patterns was a workable challenge, not a burdensome obstacle. A positive, resolute mental attitude helped a great deal. I called the health food stores in our Florida area and found one that had yeast-free breads (rice, wheat, rye) and other products that filled my needs, such as nonenriched pastas, unadulterated cereals, and nut butters. As my health improved, I realized that preparing fresh vegetables was no more of a chore than opening a package of frozen ones. The sugar cravings disappeared, and a piece of fruit soon tasted as good as any tempting, sugary dessert.

I also became more creative. Instead of jellies, I used fresh-sliced fruit, such as bananas or apples, on my nut-buttered toast. Primavera-style pasta, with fresh sautéed vegetables and olive oil instead of cream sauce, became a staple in my diet. My special treat turned out to be bananas with fresh strawberries and nuts.

A major challenge, of course, was dining out. I learned to ask many questions about how dishes were prepared, what ingredients were used, and if they could be prepared in certain ways for me. The magic word that helped was "allergies." Restaurants do not want diners having allergic reactions on their premises. I also found that the staff of most restaurants, when I persisted, was honest and eager to make my meal pleasant. The persistence was important. It is not enough to ask the servers about certain ingredients. I needed to insist that they check with the chef. Frequently I was told, "of course we only use fresh lemon on our fish, chicken . . ." only to find that lemon juice concentrate was often used in many ethnic-style dishes.

Lemon juice concentrate doesn't sound like such a bad thing, does it? But I was learning. Like many processed fruit products, lemon juice is preserved with sulfites, those ubiquitous chemicals that are primarily used to prevent discoloration in foods.

Before coming South, I had called the Food and Drug Administration (FDA) for information about food additives and preservatives. The Milwaukee office sent me a brochure titled *Food Additives* and an interesting article, "Reacting to Sulfites," that was published by the FDA public affairs staff.

I learned that "sulfites" (a salt derived from sulfurous acid) is actually a term that is applied to a variety of sulfur-based substances, and is a French variant of the word "sulfate." Sulfites include sulfur dioxide, sodium sulfite, sodium and potassium bisulfite, and sodium and potassium metabisulfite.

Sulfiting agents are used to reduce or prevent discoloration during the preparation, storage, and distribution of many foods.

Sulfites have other uses as well. Sulfur dioxide is a bleaching agent for food starches; sodium metabisulfite and sodium sulfite are used with other ingredients to prevent rust and scaling in boiler water used in making steam that will come in contact with food. Sodium sulfite and sodium metabisulfite are used in the production of cellophane for food packaging. Potassium metabisulfite, sodium bisulfite, sodium metabisulfite, and sulphur dioxide are used as sterilizing agents in wine making. Sulfites also help prevent oxidation, which can affect the potency and stability of a drug. The majority of drugs containing sulfites are intravenous injected or spray-type products. Comparatively few are oral medications.

Sulfites are placed in the "Generally Recognized As Safe" (GRAS) category by the FDA. But since the early 1980s, there has been considerable controversy and publicity about the widespread use of sulfiting agents in the nation's food supply. Between 1985 and 1990, the FDA received approximately 1,000 complaints of adverse reactions to sulfited foods, including reports of 27 deaths. After extensive investigation, the FDA acknowledged that 10 of the deaths were "probably" associated with the consumption of sulfites, 7 others were "possibly" due to sulfite consumption, and the remaining 10 were not believed to be related to sulfites.

Asthmatics are the primary population at risk for sulfite reactions. The key symptom reported by most of those affected is difficulty breathing. Other reported symptoms include wheezing, vomiting, nausea, diarrhea, unconsciousness, abdominal pain, cramps, and hives.

As a result of these complaints and reactions, some changes have been instituted. The FDA now bans the use of sulfites on fresh foods that will be eaten raw, primarily applicable to vegetables and fruits served at salad bars. Moreover, food manufacturers must now declare the presence of sulfites on product labels if the sulfite level in a finished food amounts to 10 or more parts per million. Ten parts per million, the FDA says, is the lowest detectable level of sulfites.

The FDA article included a list – which I have since learned is very limited – of common foods that use sulfiting agents. Included on the list were items prevalent in most American diets, including mine: avocado dip and guacamole, beer, cider, dried cod, fruit (fresh peeled, dried, or maraschino-type), fruit juices (and purees, and fillings), gelatin, potatoes (fresh peeled, frozen, dried, or canned), salad dressing (dry mix), relishes, salads (particularly at salad bars), sauces and gravies (canned or dried), sauerkraut, cole slaw, shellfish (fresh, frozen, canned or dried-including clams, crab, lobster, scallops, and shrimp), soups (canned or dried), vegetables (fresh peeled, frozen, canned, or dried-including fresh mushrooms), wine vinegar, wine, and wine coolers.

Later, with further investigation of sulfites, I learned more, much, much more.

As I became more sophisticated about obtaining information from the federal government, I used the Freedom of Information Act to request FDA material about sulfites not prepared for public information. In response to my request for a comprehensive list of foods and medications containing sulfites, I was sent 85 pages of the *Federal Register* and a 50-page computer printout of medications that contain sulfites. As I plodded through the *Federal Register*, I turned up some alarming tidbits: for example, some teas have "exceedingly high" sulfite levels (over 1,000 parts per million); dried apricots have sulfite levels up to 3,500 parts per million.

A "Freedom of Information" request to the FDA must be in writing to:

> Food & Drug Administration
> Freedom of Information Staff (#FI-35)
> 56 Fishers Lane
> Rockville, MD 20857

That's the easy part. In addition, you must be specific about the information requested and specify how much you are willing to pay. (The average consumer is charged for search time and copying cost – with no charge for the first two hours of search time and the first 100 pages of copying.)

My concerns grew as I delved further into the material.

"In sensitive individuals," the FDA noted, sulfites "may have serious health implications." Labeling of products with sulfites is necessary "to avoid the potential hazard of an allergic-type reaction to sulfiting agents."

My experience with sulfites over the past few years is that the problem is not the exposure to one or two foods that may contain sulfites, but the incredibly widespread use of this preservative. It is almost impossible to avoid exposure unless one stops consuming all canned, processed, bottled, or frozen foods.

Even more alarming is that labels are misleading. "No preservatives added," can mean the finished food processor has not used preservatives, but one or more of the ingredients, purchased from another source and used in the finished product, may have preservatives. There is really no way of knowing with certainty.

For example, my own investigation would not have revealed that frozen potatoes used for French fries or home fries in all restaurants are treated with sulfites to keep them from turning dark or getting black spots on them. I have yet to see sulfites listed on any cookie, cracker, or bread label, although they are used as a dough conditioner. They are also present in sweeteners, such as corn syrup. And it was only when I asked a friend who owns a restaurant that I learned the soup base, which is used in "homemade" restaurant soups, is preserved with sulfites.

As for medications, I have been healthy most of my life and rarely take medications, although I am allergic to penicillin. As I scanned the medication lists, however, I noticed Novocain. I have had continuing dental problems since childhood, often involving procedures using Novocain. As I thought back to the major dental work I have had done since I was in sixth grade, I was horrified to think of the amount of Novocain (with sulfites) that had been injected into my system.

I called my dentist, who has been taking care of my teeth since I was 20 years old, to let him know that before I needed any more work done, he would have to find Novocain or a similar product without sulfites. He checked with an oral surgeon and – wonder of wonders – there was such a product. The next time I visited him, he used the sulfite-free product, and it was the first time I did not have a physical "rush" in my system followed by heart palpitations. I didn't know that this was not the normal response to Novocain.

I thought about my pattern of feeling better during our winter breaks and experiencing a recurrence of symptoms upon our return home. I realized that a change in diet in Florida and the absence of dental procedures probably lessened my exposure to sulfites and contributed to the cessation or reduction of some fibromyalgia symptoms.

Chapter 13 contains a complete list of foods containing sulfites, plus discussion of other chemical food additives.

---

As time passed and my improvement accelerated, I occasionally "challenged" certain foods to see what my reactions might be. I found I could eat some Chinese foods if I eliminated broccoli and mushrooms and didn't use the sweet or soy sauces. There was a wonderful local Chinese restaurant in Florida that accommodated my needs and helped me experiment.

Even more difficult than eating out was dining in the homes of friends. When they asked what I could eat, no matter how I explained that "plain, unadorned food" was just fine, the food preparer, with few exceptions, would feel compelled to dress up these dishes to make them more gourmet. I clearly remember one disaster, a dinner at the home of a casual friend in Florida. "Don't make it fancy or gourmet, I can only eat simple foods," I warned her. But how was she to know that the raisins in the chicken dish contained sulfites, as do many other dried fruits; that the fruit salad she served for dessert included canned pineapple, which probably contains the highest concentration of sulfites found in any canned fruit. She had gone to a great deal of trouble to prepare a meal she thought would suit me, and I didn't want to seem unappreciative of her efforts. I ate the fruit cocktail even as I feared the consequences.

The next morning I awoke in a cold sweat, with terrible stomach pains and symptoms similar to food poisoning. I felt dizzy, as though I was going to faint, and barely managed to crawl back into bed again. Three or four hours later I slithered out of bed and returned to some feeling of normalcy.

Needless to say, I became much more careful of these dining pleasures and began to turn down invitations to eat at friends' homes. I encouraged meeting in restaurants instead, or sometimes brought my own food, like Pasta Primavera with olive oil and sautéed vegetables, rather than being deprived of a social life.

Except for the dining restrictions, our winter break was delightful. I continued stretching exercises, swimming and walking, socializing with friends, and entertaining our children and grandchildren on their visits to us. As the weeks passed, the diet and exercise seemed to work miracles. Weight disappeared at the rate of a pound a week, and I leveled off at 25 pounds less than I weighed in the fall of 1991. Joseph and I returned home. I felt great and looked trim and healthy.

# Chapter 12
# 1992: EXPANDING MY FIBROMYALGIA CIRCLE

*A courage mightier than the sun –
You rose and fought and fighting won.*
ANGELA MORGAN. *KNOW THYSELF*

Back in Milwaukee again, as spring drove out the harsh Wisconsin winter, I continued fighting battles. My health insurance company had refused reimbursement for the ELISA/ACT™ test, which cost $950.00. I appealed, and on May 7 received their final answer: "Services which are considered either investigational and/or experimental are excluded under your benefit plan." Somehow I wasn't surprised.

Considering the outcome, I have always felt the money I was willing to invest in my health was more than well spent. Since then, I have learned that the same insurance company will cover these tests for some people, but not for others, depending upon the employer's coverage.

Insurance carriers offer employers a basic package of medical benefits and other optional benefits, from which the employers can select what to include in the coverage for their employees. My ELISA/ACT™ blood test was classified as "investigational and/or experimental" and was not covered. Medicare does not cover this test either.

It remains an ironic absurdity to me that my health insurance covered untold numbers of tests and procedures that accomplished nothing, and yet would not cover a protocol that has resulted in wellness!

It is encouraging that as the ELISA/ACT™ becomes better known, an increasing number of insurance companies are covering it. To date, more than 130 health care plans will pay for this valuable test.

I was doing a great deal more than fighting losing battles against insurance companies. An interesting series of events started me on the road to one of the most exciting projects I have ever undertaken. It began with an invitation to a party on June 4, 1992, with current and past employees of the Women's Development Center at Waukesha County Technical College, where I had worked from 1980 to 1984.

It's always stimulating to get together with old friends and colleagues after a period of time and observe how people have changed. Some of the women commented about my appearance and asked what I had done to achieve this new fit and healthy look. As I shared my experiences about fibromyalgia with them, I learned that one of our co-workers, who was not at the party, had also been diagnosed with fibromyalgia. I knew I had to get in touch with her and compare notes.

Two weeks later, Karen and I talked about where she was going for help. She said she was feeling very achy and extremely tired. She told me about a medical clinic in a small town near Milwaukee, headed by a physician who seemed to have a great deal of interest in this syndrome. The clinic offered the services of a massage therapist, a chiropractor, a nutritionist, and an ongoing support group, as well as standard medical treatment.

Talking to Karen helped confirm a growing impression: I was not a medical anomaly. There were many people suffering with similar symptoms. Why shouldn't what worked for me be applicable to others? I thought about the significance of the clinical arrangement Karen had described and how my own personal experience might fit into such a framework.

Inside my head, bells were ringing and whistles were blowing. Thoughts were building – ideas tumbling over each other as I tried to conceptualize how all these puzzle pieces could fit together. I became obsessed with the idea that what seemed to be working so well for me might be helpful to others. Knowing firsthand the debilitating effects of fibromyalgia fatigue and pain, I could not walk away and say, "Oh well, I'm feeling good, it's too bad about all the others."

I understood enough about medical research to know that opinions and impressions must be backed up by scientific studies before they will be accepted by the medical community. I called the doctor associated with this clinic, told him of my experience, and naively asked if he was interested in developing a study to test the diet/nutritional supplement theory that seemed to be working so effectively for me. He was interested.

I met with the chiropractor, the nutritionist, the massage therapist, and the physician to explore the process of developing the study. I shared my experiences and we exchanged ideas. Innocently, I went home to work on a questionnaire/survey. It never occurred to me that, although these professionals had medical training, their knowledge of research techniques was limited.

In early fall, I attended a few of their fibromyalgia support group meetings, which were led by the massage therapist. I shared my experiences with this group, and we talked about their possible participation in a study. Several people expressed reservations. One of the women, a local fibromyalgia support group leader, pointed out that the study design was not scientific enough to be valid. Because of the high cost of past medical treatments that were not covered by insurance, many people in the group said they could not afford to participate if there was no funding.

While I continued to explore the idea of a study, I was fine-tuning my knowledge, rereading, researching, and summarizing the information on fibromyalgia that I had acquired from the Medical College of Wisconsin Library and other sources.

I was also testing my own health limits. Occasionally I challenged my dietary restrictions. One day, I ate a yeast-free cranberry muffin. Within a short time I was overwhelmed by such fatigue that I could barely move from my desk to lie down. After a nap, I was able to return to work. I had forgotten that cranberries were on my list of forbidden fruit.

During the summer, I also added back to my diet what I thought was an innocuous food item – a sugar-free, all-fruit jam. The label clearly stated: no preservatives, no artificial color, no artificial flavor. It seemed benign. But I couldn't help but connect it to the symptoms that were gradually reappearing. Slowly and insidiously, the pain and stiffness of fibromyalgia were returning, not to the degree I had experienced in 1991, but enough to make me know I needed to seek help.

I remembered the positive results that myofascial release therapy had achieved. I returned to Frank Fantazzi for another course of physical-therapy treatment. Again, his notes capsulated my physical condition in August of 92: Pain with rising in the morning in the right lower back; pain with turning in bed, worsening over the last few months.

He recommended muscle treatments two times per week for the next two to three weeks, and a home exercise program to strengthen the muscles that help me stand erect.

Myofascial release is a hands-on, whole-body approach for the evaluation and treatment of the human structure and is a relatively new addition to the array of skills of the physical therapist. It is generally an extremely mild and gentle form of stretching that has a profound effect upon the body tissues.

The *fascia* is a tough connective tissue system and is composed of two types of fibers – collagenous fibers, which are very tough and have little stretchability; and elastic fibers, which are stretchable.

This system extends without interruption from the top of the head to the tip of the toes. It surrounds and invades every other tissue and organ of the body, including nerves, vessels, muscle, and bone.

Because fascia spreads through all regions of the body and is interconnected, when it scars and hardens in one area (following injury, inflammation, disease, surgery, etc.), it can put tension on adjoining pain-sensitive body structures and on distant body structures as well.

After the myofascial release therapy relaxed my muscles, I quit consuming sulfites, and the tension did not return. This combination of changes clearly convinced me there was a relationship between food/chemical ingestion and the condition of my health.

In spite of the temporary setback, I still felt I was following the most promising approach to wellness. But I was also beginning to realize that despite all my research, and my vigilant reading of labels and ingredient lists, I did not have enough knowledge to totally avoid additives and preservatives. I traced this realization to the sugar-free all-fruit jam I was using. Why was it that when I stopped using this "no preservatives, no artificial color, no artificial flavor" product, the pain and fatigue disappeared? This was something that needed further investigation, and I tucked it away in my mind.

I would learn that while lemon juice was listed as an ingredient of the jam, the sulfites that were added to the lemon juice as a preservative were not. Sulfites are a much more ubiquitous part of the food supply in this country than most of us realize, and sensitivities to these chemicals may be causing low-level, subclinical health problems for many people. These people may never connect their symptoms with their diet and never be appropriately diagnosed.

The development of a research study with the clinic was moving very slowly, and looked as though it would expire without a boost of some kind. One evening, my daughter Cynthia and I brainstormed about how to overcome the obstacles I seemed to be facing. I am close to all my children, and Cynthia and I had become even closer after the death of my older daughter, Pamela.

As I shared the frustration of feeling like I was simply spinning my wheels, Cynthia wondered whether I needed a more research-oriented consultant. She suggested that I talk to Russell Jaffe at the Serammune Physicians Lab in Reston, Virginia. He is the physician who devised the ELISA/ACT™ test, which I now know has had such a major impact on my recovered health and my ideas about the effects of nutrition on wellness. Maybe he would be interested in helping with, and possibly even funding, the study.

# Part IV

## SPREADING THE WORD

## Chapter 13
## 1992-1993: CALLING IN THE EXPERTS

*Believe one who has proved it. Believe an expert.*
— VERGIL. *AENEID*, BK XI, L. 283

I already had tremendous admiration for Dr. Jaffe. He applied the basic principles of immunology and nutritional intervention to health problems, with a holistic approach that was achieving success in conditions that left less creative practitioners shaking their heads in futility. Most people who have contact with Dr. Jaffe end up using the word "genius" when they talk about this maverick scientist. But Jaffe likes to refer to himself as a "simple country doctor" and discounts any suggestion that the methods he employs are "alternative" medicine.

All we do, Dr. Jaffe says in explaining his work, is set the reset button on the control system, the neurochemical hormonal and immunologic control system.

He offers the ELISA/ACT™ test as a comprehensive and cost-effective option to the years of searching and misdiagnosis that so many people with conditions such as fibromyalgia have endured.

But his work does not stop with the diagnosis. In addition to the Serammune Physicians Lab, he runs a company called Seraphim, Inc., which manufactures and markets a comprehensive line of natural vitamins, minerals, antioxidants, and other nutritional supplements. I am still using many of these products – which are free of preservatives and additives – and feel certain they have an important role in my continuing good health.

Jaffe emphasizes, as does Dr. Norman Schwartz, the unity of the mind and body.

"You can't show me any interaction with your physical being that doesn't influence your mind," he says, "and you can't show me any interaction with your mind that doesn't influence your physical being. You just have to be aware of it, to see it in a frame of reference that's comfortable for you." (Jaffe n.d.)

With his shock of white hair and the burgundy suspenders he likes to wear, Dr. Jaffe looks a little bit like the country doctor he claims to be. Actually, he's from Albany, New York, and he received his medical training at Boston University, where he took advantage of an unusual program to receive his bachelor's degree, his medical degree and a Ph.D. at the same time. He graduated cum laude from the College of Liberal Arts with his undergraduate degree in the morning; received his Ph.D. in Biochemistry and Physiology from the Graduate School of General Medical Sciences at mid-day, and his M.D., with senior thesis honors, from the Medical School in the afternoon. This was the first time anyone at Boston University received degrees from three schools within the university in one day. He also received the J. D. Lane Award for excellence in research, as a resident, and the

Merck, Sharp, Dome research excellence award as a student.

An interest in the body's biochemical reactions to diet has been a continuing thread in his work. While at the National Institute of Health in the 1970s, he realized that his interest in the mechanism of health was something of a deviation from traditional medicine's emphasis on the mechanism of disease, and he started directing his energies toward an innovative path that he forged for himself. Today, a growing number of like-minded scientists share his philosophies and ideas and embrace the practicality of an approach that, as Dr. Jaffe describes it, provides true, lifelong, quality-of-life outcomes with crisp endpoints. ELISA/ACT™ has evolved from a test for sensitivity to just a few items, to a comprehensive panel that analyzes reactivity to almost 400 different substances. This assessment of the functionality of the human immune system is a non-invasive, cost-effective, theoretically simple means of providing information that can turn a person's life around, as I know from my own experience.

I called Dr. Jaffe and told him about the study I envisioned. He suggested that the two of us have a conference call with Dr. Schwartz to discuss some ideas about the study. We were all enthusiastic about some sort of scientific trial that would test whether eliminating substances identified as irritants by the ELISA/ACT™ would have an impact on other fibromyalgia patients, as it had on me.

During a phone conversation on November 12, we decided the study would be conducted in Milwaukee, and that I would have the task of locating the participants and facilitating the support groups that would be part of the protocol.

As it turned out, 1992 was a year of high hopes, frustrations, and learning. Some participants from the local clinic support group, described earlier, agreed to participate, if funding was available. I piqued the interest of Dr. Jaffe and the Serammune Physicians Lab to pursue this study, and started to put together what I hoped would be a nucleus of professional support. It looked as if the study might really happen.

---

But it would have to wait a few months. It was winter, and time once again for our winter get-away. I left for Florida feeling great. I maintained my weight, continued to watch my food intake, and persevered at my walking, swimming, and stretching exercises. My zest for living had returned!

It was during these months in Florida that it really began to sink in: I had achieved wellness. I was no longer fatigued, and I was going to stay well. I had energy, and could again feel excitement, wonder, and enthusiasm for life's small pleasures. I could write letters, make phone calls, and plan my work with little effort. I devoted energy to the fibromyalgia project, to my social life with my husband, friends, children, and grandchildren, and still had energy to spare. I was 60 years old and I couldn't believe how youthful I felt!

---

In April, back in Milwaukee, I received a call from Jon A. Moreshead, a physician with a specialty in family medicine. Dr. Moreshead is a clinical researcher, teacher, chemist, and agricultural researcher. He was working with Serammune Physicians Lab to document the effectiveness of diagnosing and managing delayed hypersensitivities in evoking the human healing response, even in chronic conditions generally considered degenerative and intractable.

Before working with Serammune, Dr. Moreshead had been in private practice in the Shenandoah Valley of Virginia, where he had used nutritional and holistic methods with his patients. After leaving his private practice, he adapted a method of raising turkeys on pastureland, circumventing the need for the chemical/toxic supplements, antibiotics, or growth stimulants normally used.

He told me he would be serving as the principal investigator of the ELISA/ACT™ fibromyalgia study. A stream of correspondence, telephone calls, and ideas flowed between us in the next weeks as we exchanged information and formulated questions and problems that would need to be addressed for the process to work.

The goal of the study, as Dr. Moreshead and Serammune established, was to determine the effectiveness of the ELISA/ACT™ program in the condition known as fibromyalgia, since current therapies for fibromyalgia have not addressed the underlying immune system dysfunctions as a causative factor in the symptoms of fibromyalgia.

That spring, Dr. Jaffe invited me to meet him at a conference sponsored by the American Academy of Environmental Medicine in Schaumburg, Illinois, where he was speaking.

I listened to his talk about the ELISA/ACT™ and the immune system and was tempted to stand up at the meeting and shout, "Pay attention! It really works!"

After the conference, we discussed some details about the progress of the study and what problems still needed to be resolved.

I continued to stay in touch with people who expressed an

interest in the study: the leader of a fibromyalgia support group in the Milwaukee area, a chiropractor, a massage therapist, Dr. Schwartz, and Dr. Robertson (the osteopath who worked so hard with me to keep my body mobile).

In June Dr. Moreshead was traveling in the Milwaukee area, and I arranged a dinner meeting with him at which the chiropractor, the fibromyalgia support group leader, Dr. Robertson, and I discussed the progress of the study and brainstormed ideas. A great deal of enthusiasm was generated at this meeting, and we all made a renewed commitment to our continued participation in this project.

Headway on enlisting volunteers was very slow, however. I sent packets of information to potential volunteers and received little response. I decided to cast a somewhat wider net and placed ads for volunteers in local newspapers. One community columnist wrote an item about my frustrating, but ultimately successful, search for relief from the pain of fibromyalgia. "Now Claire wants to know if the treatment she received can help others," she wrote. "Maybe Claire's pain can be your gain." (Jozwik 1993)

I also placed a short article in the medical section of our major city newspaper, the *Milwaukee Journal Sentinel,* with the headline, "Fibromyalgia Volunteers Sought for Research Study." The article briefly described the study and explained what the participants would have to do, including having their tender points verified and completing a pre- and post-study questionnaire about physical symptoms, medications, lifestyle habits, and therapies.

The publicity paid off. Although I had asked for only 20 controls, I was overwhelmed by the response from people who were eagerly hoping for something to alleviate their pain and fatigue – an alternative to the therapies that they had previously tried with little or no success. I spoke with at least 150 people, many of whom wanted to participate fully in the study. I received telephone calls from Arizona, California, New Mexico, Minnesota, and Illinois – relatives and friends of local residents who had read the brief article and contacted people they knew who were suffering from this syndrome. We wanted local subjects for the study, but I told them about what we had planned and shared my personal experience and the hope that this treatment would work for others.

Within weeks, 40 people were willing to fully participate and 29 volunteered as controls. The full participants would volunteer to have the ELISA/ACT™ blood test and modify their diets accordingly, take nutritional supplements, and make some behavioral changes such as mild exercise, meditation and/or deep breathing exercises. The control group would only complete the written reports. At the end of the study they would have the option to follow the treatment program. We were on our way!

In addition, as the work on the study continued, I communicated with every fibromyalgia contact who crossed my path. More and more, people are speaking publicly about this syndrome – one that has changed their lives in such a negative way. After years of being ignored or overlooked, newsletters about fibromyalgia are available and support groups are proliferating. I wrote letters to, or spoke with, anybody who was interested in fibromyalgia: a woman who publishes a newsletter for women suffering with chronic pain and her rheumatologist; doctors who are involved in fibromyalgia research; a congressman who professes to be interested in women's health issues; Hillary Rodham Clinton; doctors who write medical columns who are still sharing the traditional (and unhelpful) information about treatments for fibromyalgia; and *Arthritis Today* magazine in response to their article, "Fibromyalgia: Out of the Closet."

However, I learned that despite the increased discussion about fibromyalgia, there seemed to be a standard party line, and the views I had developed didn't quite fall into the acceptable range. I was totally ignored by most of the contacts I had reached out to. Even worse, the local Arthritis Society prohibited me from speaking at their sanctioned fibromyalgia support group meetings, because the treatment that worked for me did not have the approval of the Arthritis Foundation.

---

In preparation for the forthcoming study, I again contacted the local FDA office and asked for information about other additives and preservatives, such as Sodium Benzoate, Butylated Hydroxyanisole (BHA) and Butylated Hydroxytoluene (BHT), and monosodium glutamates (MSG). The secretary who assisted me also found a list of foods containing sulfites that was dated April 1991. More than 18 months after my initial request, I finally had a comprehensive list! I still wonder why the local FDA office or the Freedom of Information Agency had not initially given me this list instead of the 85 pages of the Federal Register. Oh well, what can you expect from a bureaucracy?

The FDA information I received on common foods with sulfites is presented on the following pages.

Not all manufacturers of these foods use sulfites. The amounts that are used may vary. Information from this list should be supplemented by reading the labels of packaged foods and/or contacting the manufacturer.

| FOOD CATEGORY | TYPES OF FOODS |
| --- | --- |
| **Alcoholic beverages** | Wine, beer, cocktail mixes, wine coolers |
| **Tea** | Instant tea, liquid tea concentrates |
| **Baked goods** | Cookies, crackers, mixes with dried fruits or vegetables, pie crust, pizza crust, quick crust, flour tortillas |
| **Beverage bases** | Dried citrus fruit base, bottled beverages, mixes, cider, root beer |
| **Condiments and relishes** | Horseradish, onion, and pickle relishes, pickles, olives, salad dressing mixes, wine vinegar |
| **Confections and frostings** | Brown, raw, powdered, or white sugar derived from sugar beets |
| **Dairy product analogs** | Filled milk (skim milk enriched in fat content by addition of vegetable oils) |
| **Fish and shellfish** | Canned clams, fresh, frozen, canned or dried shrimp, frozen lobster, scallops, dried cod |

| FOOD CATEGORY | TYPES OF FOODS |
| --- | --- |
| Processed fruits | Canned, bottled, or frozen fruit juices (including lemon, lime, grape, apple), dried fruit, dietetic fruit (canned, bottled or frozen), or fruit juices, maraschino cherries, glazed fruit, shredded coconut |
| Processed vegetables | Vegetable juices, canned vegetables (including potatoes), pickled vegetables (including sauerkraut, cauliflower and peppers), dried vegetables, instant mashed potatoes, frozen potatoes, potato salad |
| Gelatins, puddings fillings | Fruit fillings, flavored and unflavored gelatin, pectin, jelling agents |
| Grain products and pasta | Cornstarch, modified food starch, spinach pasta, gravies, hominy, breadings, batters, noodle/rice mixes |
| Jams and jellies | Jams and jellies |
| Plant protein products | Soy protein products |
| Snack foods | Dried fruit snacks, trail mixes, filled crackers |
| Soups and soup mixes | Canned soups, dried soup mixes |
| Sweet sauces, toppings, syrup | Corn syrup, maple syrup, fruit toppings, high-fructose corn syrup, pancake syrup, molasses |

Sodium benzoate is used as an antimicrobial agent in sweet sauces, baked goods, condiments and relishes, processed vegetables, salted margarine, seasonings and flavors, jams and jellies, fats and oils, gelatins and puddings, frosting, processed fruit, imitation dairy products, gravies, alcoholic and nonalcoholic beverages, fruit ices, milk products, soft candy, frozen dairy products, instant coffee and tea, meat products, breakfast cereals, hard candy, and cheese.

BHA, and a chemically similar compound, BHT, are antioxidants used for more than 40 years to retard rancidity in a wide array of food products containing fats and oils, as well as in certain processed meat products. They are both direct additives and indirect additives put into defoaming agents, food packaging materials, adhesives, and lubricants that come into contact with food.

BHA and BHT generally are used in breakfast cereals, chewing gum, convenience foods, vegetable oils, shortening, potato flakes, enriched rice, potato chips, and candy – to name some. Their ability to intercept oxygen before it gets to fat molecules is what makes them effective in keeping food from becoming rancid.

Monosodium glutamate (MSG) has been used for many years as a flavor enhancer for a variety of foods prepared at home, in restaurants, and by food processors. The substance has become controversial because some people believe they suffer allergic-type reactions when they consume MSG. Because of MSG's common use in Chinese cuisine, these reactions have become known popularly as "Chinese restaurant syndrome."

The FDA has studied adverse reaction reports and other data concerning MSG's effects for many years. The agency believes that sensitive people can have mild and transitory reactions in some circumstances when they consume significant amounts of MSG (such as would be found in heavily flavor-enhanced foods). Asians have used MSG as a flavor enhancer for at least 2,000 years in the form of a broth made with the types of seaweed known as sea tangle. Today, MSG is manufactured by a fermentation process using starch, sugar beets, sugar cane, or molasses.

MSG, as sold in grocery stores, is a fine, white crystal substance, similar in appearance to salt or sugar. It does not have a distinct taste of its own. Precisely how MSG works to "wake up" or enhance the flavor of foods is not fully understood. Many Western scientists believe that MSG stimulates taste receptors in the tongue, while their Eastern counterparts believe the chemical has a unique fifth basic taste – beyond salty, sweet, sour, and bitter – that they call "unami," derived from the Japanese word meaning "deliciousness."

A controlled study was conducted in 1972 by Richard A. Kenney, Ph.D., of George Washington University Medical Center, Washington, D.C. Dr. Kenney's study used placebos and orally administered MSG in a representative sample of people. The study showed that one-third of those tested experienced symptoms when given large doses of MSG, but, at amounts normally consumed with food, almost none did. In fact, some people who claimed to be sensitive to MSG reacted similarly when exposed to the placebo.

Scientists' concerns are not related to consumption of foods that naturally contain glutamates – a major building block of many proteins such as cheese, meat, peas, mushrooms, and milk. Their concern, rather, is that a diet extremely high in MSG used as a flavor enhancer could result in acute elevation of glutamate in the blood. Hypothetically, this could cause over-stimulation of portions of the brain, adversely affecting the central nervous system and possibly leading to brain injury. However, no scientific evidence has surfaced to support the hypothesis that MSG, consumed at levels found in food products, can cause brain injury.

The information regarding MSG came directly from the Food and Drug Administration files in 1993. Of the participants in the 1994 fibromyalgia study, 42½ percent tested sensitive to monosodium glutamate (MSG). Read on and weep regarding the latest update on MSG provided by NoMSG.

A grass roots organization, NoMSG (National Organization Mobilized to Stop Glutamate), has been created to educate consumers regarding the dangers of monosodium glutamate and the ways in which it is hidden, to encourage MSG-free products, to support MSG-sensitive individuals, and to promote independent MSG research.

> MSG is a drug and neurotransmitter, a nerve transmission substance. The ever-expanding use of MSG causes great concern in the medical profession because it stimulates brain cell activity. MSG "tricks" the brain into thinking the food you are eating tastes good. Manufacturers can use inferior ingredients and thus make the product seem tastier. MSG intolerance is not an allergic reaction but a powerful drug reaction.
>
> These common reactions can include headaches, migraines, stomach upset, fatigue, nausea and vomiting, diarrhea, irritable bowel syndrome, asthma attacks, shortness of breath, anxiety or panic attacks, heart palpitations, partial paralysis, heart-attack-like

symptoms, balance difficulties, mental confusion, mood swings, depression, behavior disorders (especially in children and teens), allergy-type symptoms – skin rashes, runny nose, bags under the eyes, flushing and mouth lesions.

MSG in its pure form must be labeled. However, when it is added as an ingredient of another substance it need not be listed on the label. The earlier these "hidden" substances appear on a list of ingredients, the more likely they are to contain MSG. NoMSG advises avoiding all possible sources.

Definite sources of MSG include: hydrolyzed protein, sodium caseinate or calcium caseinate, autolyzed yeast or yeast extract, gelatin.

Possible substances harboring MSG: textured protein; carrageenan or vegetable gum; seasonings or spices; flavorings or natural flavorings; smoke flavorings for chicken, beef and pork; prepackaged bouillon, broth, or stock; barley malt, malt extract or malt flavoring; whey protein, whey protein isolate or concentrate; soy protein, soy protein isolate, or concentrate; soy sauce or extract. (NO MSG 1999)

This list is periodically updated by the networking membership of NoMSG, who also suggest elimination of aspartame and sulfites from the diet. The list is not all inclusive, because new labeling deceptions are continually invented to confound the consumer. (More information on NoMSG is provided in the Resources section at the end of this book.)

In August, I attended a meeting at which Steve Davis, a

public affairs specialist from the FDA Milwaukee office, spoke about the new Nutrition Facts labels that would soon be used on all processed foods, providing information about calories, fat, sodium, carbohydrates, cholesterol, potassium, protein, etc. During the question period following the talk, I asked Mr. Davis why labels did not indicate additives such as sulfites. Wanting to avoid the question, he said he would speak with me after the program. At that time he asked me to write him a letter detailing my experience with sulfites.

I wrote the letter on August 25, 1993; it was received by his office on August 30, and forwarded to Linda R. Tollefson of the Center for Food Safety and Applied Nutrition in Washington, D.C. I have since learned that complaint letters such as mine, when received by government offices, are identified by topics and lumped together with all other similar letters. They are then weighed. When the preponderance of this topic is sufficient, attention will be given to the subject.

---

Meanwhile, Patricia Deuster replaced Dr. Moreshead as principal investigator of the study. Dr. Deuster has a doctorate in nutritional sciences and biochemistry. She is currently an associate professor in the Department of Military and Emergency Medicine at the Uniformed Services University of the Health Sciences in Bethesda, Maryland. She is director of research and director of the human performance laboratory. Dr. Deuster has written over 70 scientific articles, several book chapters, and numerous articles used by physicians and other health professionals.

Dr. Deuster has given hundreds of presentations on nutrition, chronic disease, and sports nutrition, and recently completed a book on nutrition and performance for the Navy. Her current research includes work on nutrition and exercise in patients with fibromyalgia and rheumatoid arthritis, and nutritional interventions to accelerate the healing process and improve human performance. She also applied her considerable scientific investigative skills to the areas of food sensitivities, environmental pollutants and health, and herbal medicines.

Dr. Deuster and I communicated about final details of the study. She was interested in the fine points: the supplements I was taking, the procedures I would be using for checking tender points, the final format of the questionnaires, the availability of support groups, and the timeline for the process. I envisioned that the medical records release could be completed in November, the tender point checks done by the end of January, blood drawn for the ELISA/ACT™ and results returned from the lab by the end of March, and the start of all diets, supplements, and support groups by April of 1994.

There was no way to foresee the pitfalls yet to come, so, packing my typewriter and all papers relating to the fibromyalgia study, Joseph and I left for our winter stay in Florida.

# Chapter 14
# 1994: MOVING FORWARD

*Attempt the end, and never stand to doubt,*
*Nothing's so hard but search will find it out.*
— ROBERT HERRICK. *SEEK AND FIND*

I was still in Florida when I received the completed format of the study from Dr. Deuster. I looked over the material with excitement. All the details were finalized. We were ready to roll.

I sent 71 packets of information to the participants and controls. The packets included a variety of documents. The Volunteer Agreement, under the imprimatur of Health Studies Collegium, Dr. Jaffe's nonprofit research arm, explained that the "goal of the present project is to determine the effectiveness of the ELISA/ACT™ program in the condition known as fibromyalgia."

It continued with an explanation of the underlying philosophy of the study.

> Current therapies for fibromyalgia have not addressed the possiblity that a disturbance in your immune system

plays a causative role in fibromyalgia, nor what health benefits will result when the body begins to repair those disturbances. This study will begin to address the immune system issue by offering nutritional and lifestyle modifications based on how your blood reacts to over 300 [at that time] foods and chemicals it may be exposed to. Once these reactive substances are identified and removed from your body, we expect the repair process will begin. (Deuster 1996)

The "Health Symptoms and Survey Prequestionnaire" gathered information about the participant's medical history, particularly relating to fibromyalgia. Baseline symptoms evaluated before beginning the protocol would be used to evaluate the degree of dysfunction in both groups, and the subjects would serve as their own controls when testing the effectiveness of the program individually.

In addition to specific questions about location, severity, and nature of pain, the questionnaire included a detailed mild-to-severe self-assessment (rated on a scale of 1 to 100) of 26 different symptoms. These included the wide array of conditions we fibromyalgia patients had come to know all too well over the years: from sleep disturbances to cold hands and feet, from migraine headaches to irritable bowel syndrome, from blurred vision to bladder spasms to premenstrual syndrome. This form would be filled out twice more – three months later in the middle of the study, and at its conclusion in six months.

The participants were also asked to provide information about how much they had spent on their medical care for fibromyalgia over the past year.

They were given detailed explanations of the process for tender point checks and blood draws, personal code numbers, instructions for receiving the nutritional supplements, and the cost to participate. Those participating in the control group were given code numbers and the process for tender point checks. They were requested to complete the paperwork and to attend designated support groups.

We had not heard about independent funding for the study, and Dr. Jaffe decided the Serammune Physicians Lab would perform the blood tests at the cost of the co-payment, as if all participants had insurance that covered the ELISA/ACT™. He also agreed that the supplements would be provided at 50 percent of retail cost. All tender point checks would be performed by Dr. Robertson at no charge to participants or controls.

The structure was in place, but the unpredictability of human nature was not factored in.

As the months passed in the sunny south, weather reports from Wisconsin were dismal. It turned out to be one of the coldest and snowiest winters in the past five years, preventing many in the study from making and/or keeping appointments for tender point checks and blood draws. One postponement was the result of a heart attack and subsequent bypass surgery.

When we returned to Milwaukee, I contacted all the volunteers to discuss their status in the study and to answer any questions. The reports were somewhat discouraging. Of the original 71 volunteers, 36 decided to drop for various reasons: one because she developed diabetes; some because even with the reduced costs, they could not afford to participate; others because their personal physicians discouraged them;

several because they were moving out of the state; and a few for no reasons they cared to share with me.

As the word spread that there were openings in the study, people again called to volunteer. Some who had originally volunteered to be controls asked to participate in the full study because nothing had changed in their medical conditions in the seven months since they first contacted me. Instead of all the participants starting on April 1, Dr. Deuster extended the starting date of the study two months, to June 1, to accommodate the late starters. On that date, we had 46 participants and 20 people in the control group. All participants were informed that I would be facilitating support groups each Thursday evening, alternating between the participant and control groups.

---

Our first meeting with all the participants occurred on April 7, 1994. It felt like opening night of a play – complete with excitement and butterflies for me! We briefly introduced ourselves and, with no particular plan in mind, I asked for questions. As the questions poured out, I could hear the fear and panic that I, too, had experienced initially when confronted with the ELISA/ACT™ test results and the reality of the extensive changes that were necessary to repair and rebuild my compromised immune system.

I explained what I had learned about the complexities of the human immune defense and repair system – how it is constantly challenged by substances in our environment, such as food and chemicals, that can have an impact on our overall health and well-being. This defense and repair system can be overwhelmed by substances that the immune system (white blood cells) adversely reacts to, and this chain of events – exposure to substances and reaction of the white blood cells – may increase our susceptibility to infectious disease and/or hypersensitivity or allergic reactions. Immune overload dysfunction can be manifested in recurrent infections and/or in chronic inflammatory and/or autoimmune syndromes such as fibromyalgia.

Two hours flew by. I listened, answered questions, shared my experiences and the encouraging improved health results I had attained by following the dietary changes recommended by the ELISA/ACT™. I assured everyone over and over that compliance with the regimen could perhaps work for them as well.

Not only were participants advised to eliminate substances that were identified as irritants for them, but they were also to strengthen their diets with therapeutically targeted supplementation. The nutritional supplements were considered an important component of the protocol. While trials of the supplements alone had not proved to be very beneficial for fibromyalgia patients, Dr. Jaffe felt it was important they be introduced to stimulate repair at the same time the cycle of immunologic damage is broken.

---

Our subsequent support group meetings were more structured. Personal research tasks, which would be helpful to others in the group, were assigned. The focus of the meetings became that of helping each other with ideas and information about ways to reduce exposure to the various harmful substances – toxic minerals, such as mercury, lead, cadmium, aluminum; environmental chemicals such as toluene, xylene, dibutyl phthalate and malleic anhydride; nutritional additives and preservatives such as aspartame, BHA, food coloring, MSG, saccharine, sodium benzoate and sulfites. Copies of the FDA food preservatives information and the Candida albicans control diet were distributed to those who needed them.

At some meetings we discussed the practicalities of this new regimen in our lives – what substitutes could be made for dairy products, yeast breads, wheat or corn, synthetic detergents and soaps; where to shop for the least contaminated foods; how to read and interpret labels; how to determine whether labels were accurate; and how soon to reintroduce the avoided foods.

One participant researched where to purchase "gas" masks. These, used to prevent inhalation of toxic paint fumes, can also be helpful for people sensitive to fumes of petroleum fuels (gasoline). They can be used when pumping gas at the filling station, when stalled in traffic, or even when just walking through parking lots.

For those people in the study who suffered from seasonal affective disorder (SAD), the test information handbook recommended a dichromatic or green light. SAD is a depressive disorder in which patients react to the shorter days and longer nights of midwinter. A person sits four to six feet from the face of a green light for 20 minutes, twice daily. This is typically done in the morning and early evening. During this time s/he can perform other activities such as deep breathing, relaxation, guided imagery, range of motion exercises, and reading, since it is not necessary to look directly at the light.

These dichromatic lights help modify moods and reduce

symptoms. We found a local source for the socket-clamp light holders and bulbs. Buying them at Fleet Farm was less costly than ordering them from catalogs.

For those people in the study who reacted to chemical compounds such as pesticides, metallics, and mercury, we shared information about the use of a Clorox bath for fruits and vegetables. This removes sprays, bacteria, fungus, and metallics, and seems to help people with compromised immune systems.

**Treatment**
- Use ½ teaspoon of Clorox bleach to one gallon of water.
- Thin-skinned fruits, berries, and leafy vegetables require 5-10 minutes in the bath. Root vegetables and heavy skinned fruits require 15-20 minutes.
- Remove from the bath and place into a clean, fresh water bath for 15-20 minutes. Food is now ready for further preparation.

**Cautions**
- Make a fresh bath for each group you are treating.
- Don't use Clorox on mushrooms.
- Leave skins on food.

**Advantages**
- Fruits and vegetables will keep much longer.
- Wilted food will return to fresh crispness.
- Many parasites and their eggs will be destroyed.
- Your food will look better and the flavor will be greatly enhanced, as if fresh from a garden.

In an independent test done in 1983, Sommer-Frey Laboratories in Milwaukee found that peaches put through the Clorox bath were significantly lowered in mercury contamination – from 0.011 ppm to 0.003 ppm (parts per million). using 1/2 teaspoon of Clorox bleach to one gallon of water.

There are two other commercial products available– Fruit Wash and Dr. Bronner's Salsuds – through health food stores such as the Outpost in Milwaukee. Follow the directions carefully. Do not use any of these washes if you are sensitive to any of the ingredients.

Much of our discussion in the support group meetings centered on how to do an ascorbate or Vitamin C flush, loading the system with Vitamin C. (Consult with your ELISA/ACT™ physician regarding this process.) Vitamin C promotes cellular healing and increases resistance to viral infections. Almost all animals and plants synthesize their own Vitamin C, except guinea pigs, monkeys, and humans. The first two animals eat mostly fresh, Vitamin C-rich foods. Humans, in this modern world, do not. Because of premature food harvesting, artificial ripening, and processing, many of our foods contain less and less Vitamin C.

Glucose and Vitamin C are similar structurally, and it may be that some sugar cravings represent a need for Vitamin C. Taking Vitamin C is often helpful for those cravings. In addition, Vitamin C has countless important functions within an organism and within a cell – related to cell repair and division, energy production, and antioxidant effects which neutralize toxins.

There are many difficulties with a study such as this and with the ELISA/ACT™ program in general. It takes a great deal of motivation to adhere to the rigid dietary restrictions – especially when friends, relatives, and what appears to be the rest of the world – are all chowing down on burgers, fries, cakes, pies, sundaes, and even healthy foods that you have been prohibited from eating. This can be very discouraging.

Until the diet and nutritional supplements begin to take effect, one feels as though there is nothing to eat, and very little purpose to the restrictions. When we discussed compliance with diet restrictions, one participant replied with the plaintive grievance of so many of us: I have to eat something! The regimen is particularly difficult for people who live in small towns without a health food store that carries yeast-free breads or organic fruits and vegetables. The pain and fatigue of fibromyalgia can make the extra effort necessary to purchase these items almost more than one can cope with.

During the course of the study, we saw a number of phenomena. For several months, some participants were reluctant to talk about their improving health because they felt it was a fluke and would not last. Others weren't convinced the process would work for them at all. Some participants, eager to test their new feeling of wellness, reintroduced the allergens too early and had temporary setbacks. To again experience the symptoms at their worst was a valuable reminder of why they were enrolled in the study. One woman described the process of her healing as similar to peeling an onion. This simile had meaning for many in the study. As the layers of symptoms came away, others were revealed. Sometimes, it was only as the toxins were removed that secondary conditions became more obvious and could be treated.

As the months flew by, it became clear to me that the participants could be segregated into three groups:

- Those who worked very hard at complying with the ELISA/ACT™ protocol of diet restrictions, reduced toxic chemical exposure, nutritional supplements, and moderate exercise. They were showing marked improvement in their health.
- Those who were attempting compliance, but were not improving.
- Those who seemed unable or unwilling to comply.

Several in the first group were reluctant to share their observations about the improvement in their health. They needed to be sure that what they were experiencing was not going to disappear. Some of them told the group it was their friends and families who first noted subtle changes in their postures and signs of increased energy.

However, some participants were improving sufficiently to share their experiences. Their recovery could not be denied or explained away. For some, going on the Candida albicans control diet, a yeast-free diet created by Dr. William G. Crook, author of *The Yeast Connection*, resulted in a weight loss of 35 to 50 pounds. Others spoke of renewed energy that they hadn't had in 10 to 15 years. One person gained 25 pounds which, although he was trying, he hadn't been able to do for several years because of serious digestive problems. He attributed these problems to eating fruits and vegetables contaminated with pesticides.

As one woman described her improvement, "My muscles, which had felt like they were hard and cemented, were finally softening as though they were 'ripping apart.'" Some people did not speak of how they had improved, but they were observably better in physical appearance and demeanor. Their skin tones looked healthier, they were more neatly dressed, they smiled more often, and occasionally even expressed some humor, which was rare at this stage of the study.

Others, however, experienced difficulty with the program in general, including an inability to consume the nutritional supplements. Some participants had additional problems that needed to be resolved, which became more obvious when there was no noticeable improvement after several months.

Those who were complying, but not showing improvement, were encouraged to contact Dr. Robertson, Dr. Deuster, or Dr. Jaffe. Dr. Jaffe suggested that we hold a telephone conference for our meeting on June 23.

Eight participants who were having the most difficulties joined Dr. Robertson at 6:30 P.M. for what was supposed to be a one-hour consultation to discuss their personal medical problems with Dr. Jaffe. The dialogue continued well past the appointed time, and I invited the participants who had arrived for the regularly scheduled support group to listen to the discussion. At 9:40 P.M., Dr. Jaffe finally said his goodbyes, and the participants left with information and the assurance that help was available.

Dr. Robertson continued to work closely with Dr. Jaffe to help the participants who needed further testing and treatments. These additional tests resulted in the diagnosis of such problems as adrenal dysfunction, reflex sympathetic dystrophy, hypothyroidism and intestinal parasites and amoebas. One amoebae called Endolimax has been found to be associated with reactive arthritis.

As the layers of the onion peeled away in patient after patient, other conditions came to light. One participant had to move to a new home because the tight construction of her present home prevented outside air exchange, resulting in a major problem with molds and mildew. Continued gastrointestinal problems revealed one person had a cryptosporidium (a water-based parasite) condition, a hold-over from the outbreak in Milwaukee's water system in 1993.

The onion-peeling process also made it possible to connect certain foods with specific reactions. Just as I could identify white potatoes with depression, and sulfites with generalized aches, pains, and fatigue, someone else identified barley with pain on the bottom of her feet. A third person identified sugar consumption with excessive anger and acting out, and sulfites with lower back pain. Another identified organophosphates with gastrointestinal distress.

As a result of additional tests recommended by Dr. Jaffe, another participant, who also has multiple sclerosis, was diagnosed with seven other immune disorders.

Some of the participants, however, were lax about completing their three- and six-month progress reports. A few who started late had not reached the six-month point and could not yet complete those reports. A bit of nagging helped, but some reports were never completed.

I was learning how difficult it could be to transfer my enthusiasm to others, but I was also learning that persistence pays off. Soon it would be time for Dr. Deuster to analyze the mountain of paperwork that would determine whether our efforts had produced the desired results.

Joseph's 75th birthday was in October, and 21 of our children and grandchildren gathered to celebrate. It has been the anticipation and joy of these celebrations of life which have given us the courage to cope with, as Shakespeare wrote, "the slings and arrows of outrageous fortune." Everybody enjoyed what turned out to be the last time so many of us were together.

On the way to Florida that year, we stopped in Virginia, to visit the Serammune Physicians Lab. I wanted to see the lab and better understand the work that was done there. Set in the suburbs of northern Virginia, just outside of Washington, D.C., the unassuming brick building gives little clue to the magnitude of the work that goes on inside. I observed the lab technicians painstakingly testing tubes of blood for reactions to the more than 300 purified foods, preservatives, chemicals, and minerals encompassed in the ELISA/ACT™. I met many of the staff who had so diligently coped with the confusion and turmoil of our complicated study. It was wonderful to put faces to the voices I had been in contact with for so many months.

# Chapter 15
## THE STORIES OF OTHERS

*Diet cures more than doctors.*
— A. B. CHEALES. *PROVERBIAL FOLK-LORE*. NO. 82

Illness, particularly with a disease as difficult to pin down and as unpredictable as fibromyalgia, can be an isolating experience. Part of what has been so reassuring and encouraging about my personal journey toward health has been the discovery that I am not alone in this struggle.

Five of the participants in the fibromyalgia study volunteered to share their histories here to illustrate both the commonalities and individualized courses of fibromyalgia. These are their stories, told in their own words.

I begin with Karen Kilmer – it was learning about her diagnosis of fibromyalgia that stimulated me to begin the study. Karen and I had worked together at the Waukesha County Technical College. She is a warm, friendly, and helpful person, well-suited to her position as an administrative assistant. When I asked her about her fibromyalgia experience, she graciously shared the information.

### KAREN KILMER

Karen is in her 30s, married, and lives with her husband and son in New Berlin, Wisconsin. She has a big-boned body and, from my 5'1" perspective, is tall. At the start of the study she was overweight. Six months later and 30 pounds lighter, she was more attractive than I had ever seen her. Her soft blond hair is shiny, her cheerful face glows with good health, and her body curves in all the right places.

### Karen's Story

About five years ago, in 1989, I started noticing feelings I had never experienced before. I ached and was extremely tired and extremely stiff when I got up in the mornings. It was so bad that I needed to hang onto the walls to walk until the stiffness wore off. Many times on my ten-mile drive to work, I came close to renting a motel room and going to sleep. I attributed these feelings to my age [30s] and to my being overweight.

About two and a half years ago I went to the doctor's office for treatment for a sinus infection. I usually did this a couple of times a year. However, even as an antibiotic knocked out the infection, my headaches kept coming back. The doctor told me that my infection was cleared up but the headaches were from tension. He suggested that I try massage therapy. I did, but that was probably the worst month of my life, spent in pain and fatigue. The pain was so bad that sometimes I would just lie on the massage table in tears.

After discussion with both, my chiropractor and my osteopath diagnosed me with fibromyalgia. Because I also had arthritis on my spine, they wanted to stabilize that before treating the fibromyalgia. In time, between the chiropractor and massage therapy, I was feeling better, but still not as well as I wanted.

Then I heard about this study through a friend of mine [Claire] who had been on the ELISA/ACT™ elimination program for two years. She explained that with the elimination of certain foods, along with exercise, she felt 99 percent improved. She wanted to form a study group to research this idea and write a book.

At this time, I've been on the program for approximately five and one-half months, and I really do notice a difference. My energy level is up, and the pain and fatigue are minimal. I feel that I have joined the human race again.

### Barbara Leonard

Barbara is a young grandmother in her 50s. Her body is the kind that grandchildren love to cuddle up to – soft and inviting. Because of her almost total disability, she is living with one of her married children and grandchildren in Kenosha, Wisconsin. She is quiet-spoken, and my impression of her is that she is a private person. Her fibromyalgia symptoms prevent her from participating in even simple social pleasures, such as dining with friends or attending a movie.

### Barbara's Story

I became totally disabled October 2, 1990. No one could ever forget the day their life as they knew it ended. I spent October, November, and then December thinking at any moment I would get up and resume my active, happy life – a life that was filled with work, family, friends, and fun. It wasn't to be.

Those months, and the following four years, were filled with one doctor, hospital, test, and therapy after another. I did not get better, only much worse. I was told by various "experts" that I was depressed (of course I was – I wanted my life back); that I needed mental health therapy (perhaps I had been abused as a child – NOT!!). Maybe I had heart, circulatory, bowel, stomach, brain, bone, muscle, or who-knows-what problems. The point of this long-suffering list is: until I joined this fibromyalgia study group, I had been given a pharmacy full of medications to mask, or otherwise mute, all of the fevers, signs, and symptoms of my endless list and had not improved by as much as 10 percent from October 1990.

I was a little skeptical that food and/or chemical sensitivities could be creating such havoc with my system. But I was desperate and decided to play along. Thankfully, my skepticism was unfounded, and I have been proven wrong.

I had never been plagued with what I thought of as typical allergies. As a child, I had a few "minor" things that caused reactions I didn't really pay much attention to – strawberries, iodine, aspirin, penicillin – but I seemed to tolerate even these as I grew older.

Within one week of eliminating the foods that the ELISA/ACT™ showed I reacted to, I could feel an improvement. I no longer felt that my skin was unable to contain my body, and that my head was "fluffy." The irritable bowel symptoms began to subside, and I no longer felt jumpy all day. For the next three months, I could see a gradual improvement in my general feeling of well-being. My sleeping patterns improved, and I was once again able to add some simple numbers together and come up with the correct answer! What a rush!!

My brain was functioning the way it should. Thoughts once again began to flow instead of starting and stopping with some unknown will of their own. The hallucinatory nightmares I was experiencing have all but disappeared, so the quality of my sleep is much better. Of course, I feel more in control and better able to function. My pain is greatly diminished and can be kept under control by staying away from my "bad foods."

I have discovered that each food I reacted to has its own place in the body that it "hits." Barley will always give me irritable bowel syndrome and pains in the bottom of my foot. Food coloring brings on itching, hives (if I eat enough), and red, hot hands. Caffeine makes me "buzz" and tomatoes cause blisters in my mouth – to name just a few reactions I get.

It's no wonder that for four years I thought I was losing my mind. With such a cornucopia of symptoms and body systems involved, I'm amazed I wasn't committed somewhere.

After six months I'm not completely well, but I do feel better than I have for years. I don't know if this is the complete answer to all of my health problems, but I am 100 percent positive that I have improved, and that I will continue on the road to complete recovery. For the first time in years I have hope that there is really an end to this baffling "thing" I am recovering from. There could be no greater gift than that.

## Michelle Krawczyk

Michelle is a 42-year-old wife and mother of two children. She lives in Menomonee Falls, Wisconsin, a small town northwest of Milwaukee. She is vivacious, has a small-boned wiry build and is able to share, in detail, her body awareness. At present, she is an unemployed paralegal on disability assistance.

### Michelle's Story

My story begins after the birth of my daughter, Jaimee, in 1983. I was in excellent health before my pregnancy. During pregnancy, I experienced repeated bouts of bronchitis and upper respiratory ailments. Jaimee was born full-term, but with a seizure disorder.

My husband is a Vietnam veteran who was repeatedly exposed to Agent Orange. Research articles I have from the Association of Birth Defect Children indicate that Agent Orange exposure to the babies prenatally can cause serious immune dysfunction and behavior and attention problems. Both of my children have been diagnosed with attention deficit disorder, and Jaimee also has neurological impairments and has had severe allergies since birth. She had the ELISA/ACT™ test done while I was participating in this study and has shown remarkable improvement by adhering to the suggested restrictions.

After Jaimee's birth I experienced fatigue so severe after eating meals I could not function My severe respiratory ailments such as bronchitis and massive sinus infections continued.

Nothing helped until a nutritionist suggested that I was suffering from a problem – Candida albicans, a yeast-like fungus that exists in the intestinal tract and can become unbalanced. I started treatment with nystatin, an antibiotic and fungicide, and remember feeling like a miracle had taken place. The fatigue became bearable, although I never did have the energy I had before I had my children. From 1983 to 1988, I continued to battle my yeast problem by using nystatin and trying to avoid bread and other foods that would aggravate the yeast.

I was very active. I played in a racquetball league once a week and took an aerobics class twice a week. Then one day in 1988, at the age of 34, I rolled over in bed one morning and heard a loud crunch in my neck. I couldn't turn my head for several weeks. I was treated by a chiropractor for six months, but as soon as I discontinued the treatment the pain returned.

From there I sought help from an orthopedic specialist, who could find nothing wrong except a compression of nerves and arteries in my chest, which he called "thoracic outlet syndrome." He referred me for physical therapy. When I discontinued the physical therapy, the pain all came back.

I lost my job as a paralegal because I told my boss I could no longer do the physical aspects of the work, which involved a lot of driving to the courthouse, waiting in long lines with a heavy briefcase and massive caseloads. My ability to concentrate was decreasing every day.

I sought the help of a neurologist because of a burning pain between my shoulder blades. He suspected a TMJ-type problem and referred me to the hospital for evaluation. I was prescribed more physical therapy.

Then, because of jaw and left ear problems, I was referred to another specialist. The splint therapy the specialist prescribed caused me more pain than I had started with, so I discontinued his care after four weeks and sought the help of another jaw specialist. Despite treatment for nine months, I experienced increasing jaw pain and headaches.

I applied for disability assistance and won my case with the Social Security Administration in September, 1991. Because of daily incapacitating headaches, two years later, in May, 1993, I had an automobile accident. My spine and jaw were pulled off 14 millimeters to the left. After much chiropractic therapy, my spine was finally in alignment. My jaw problems were resolved in December of 1993, and I no longer needed to wear a jaw splint.

I was first diagnosed with fibromyalgia by my jaw doctor in 1992, and by Dr. Allan Robertson (to whom I went for muscle balancing work) in 1993.

My condition was so severe during this time that when my physical therapist asked me to move my body from side to side, I could only move about one-half inch in either direction. I couldn't lift my arms over my head to reach for anything without pulling my neck out of position, and I needed daily rest because I was so exhausted. The pain was constant and my state of mind was extremely irritable. I wanted to lie down by 4:00 P.M. every afternoon, up until the date I started this study. From 1991 until 1992, I had given up any kind of exercise, following the advice of my jaw doctor who said I was straining already strained muscles.

Being in the study has been a remarkable experience for me. Lo and behold, on my list of delayed hypersensitivity reactions were Candida albicans and brewers yeast. This yeast problem had plagued me for 11 years. I also had delayed hypersensitivity reactions to beef, tomato, lead, cherries, berries, aspartame, BHA, SDS, herbal tea, cinnamon, tea, chocolate, acetaminophen, cloves, and more.

Within the first two months of the study, I lost 20 pounds. My doctor told me the muscle swelling in my back was diminished, and his visible examination of my neck found it at least an inch narrower on each side. I experienced (and am still experiencing) the sensation of "ripping" of tight muscles, which leaves me with greater range of motion, less restriction of my neck, fewer headaches, and a lighter feeling. The most pronounced effect I have noticed is my increase in energy. I have been up until midnight more nights than I can count. I am doing social things I haven't been able to do for many years, like sitting through a movie or eating out at a restaurant. I have even chaperoned my children's field trips and gone on bus and car trips without excruciating pain.

My ultimate goal is to wake up in the morning and be able to go to work, or anywhere for that matter, without having to go to the YMCA to exercise, and to enjoy a day free of pain, headache, and muscle tightness.

## GLENN PATTY

Glenn is a 40-year-old man, tall, with dark hair and a slender build. He is married, has two daughters, and works for Chrysler in Kenosha, Wisconsin, as a machine tool technician, repairing machinery. Friends and family would describe him as personable, fun, a good story teller, and a workaholic. He is a considerate man who chauffeured other study participants to the support group meetings twice a month.

**Glenn's Story**

I was about 14 when I noticed subtle changes in my health. I felt kind of spacey and had red eyes. I went to see a doctor and he said nothing was wrong. That was the start of a long road from doctor to doctor, trying to get some answers. By the time I was 16, I started getting stomachaches and diarrhea. I told the doctor that it seemed certain foods would cause my problems. He said he had never heard of a problem like this before.

When I was 18, I started losing my concentration and self-confidence and generally felt lousy. I went to the same doctor again and told him I wanted to see an allergist. I did so, and told him I had food allergies. He did a Rast test (a test for immediate allergic reactions) and nothing showed up.

I went back to the doctor. He put me through many tests, including upper GI, lower GI, proctoscopes, x-rays and biopsies. There were no results. I was still complaining, so he gave me various medications. Still no results. The doctor kept telling me there was nothing wrong, and I had to live with it. I can't begin to tell you what it was like, living every day miserable. I can only describe my symptoms as a cross between food poisoning and the flu.

After my doctor died, my new doctor said he thought I needed more fiber, so I took Metamucil. At that time I discovered I was allergic to psyllium and food coloring. He redid all the tests my previous doctor had taken, and found nothing. I went to see an intestinal specialist, who did the same tests again and found nothing.

Every trip to a doctor was getting more and more frustrating. I had a doctor who thought I needed a psychiatrist, an allergist who believes a scratch test is the only way to detect food allergies and a gastroenterologist who doesn't know anything about food intolerances.

After I lost 40 pounds in six months, I decided to take my health into my own hands. I knew intuitively that my symptoms were being caused by something in the food I was eating, or the food itself. My muscles and joints were tight, my arthritis was bad, I had diarrhea and weight loss. This was hard on my family, too, as I was not my real self.

Through research and luck, I determined that my immune system was being compromised. I also got a call from someone who was having similar experiences. She told me of a study going on for people with fibromyalgia. I went to Complete Health Services in Milwaukee to see Dr. Allan Robertson. I was tested and found to have some symptoms of fibromyalgia. I was also tested for delayed reactions to 300 food and chemical items. This test confirmed that I was allergic to 21 foods, or groups, including dairy, food colorings, tomatoes, and many more.

At this time I was given supplements as part of the study and told to avoid the foods to which I had a reaction. I couldn't tolerate these supplements, so I have gone out and purchased individual supplements of my own. I seemed to tolerate these much better. I also had an immediate reaction test (as opposed to the ELISA/ACT™ delayed reaction test) for 190 foods, and found that I was allergic to eggs, wheat, psyllium, etc.

When I brought these test results to the doctors in my insurance plan, I met nothing but resistance. Apparently, the health insurance industry does not believe in food allergies. I believe if this problem had been caught early, I might have avoided the misery I have experienced for 25 years.

I've written to the insurance commissioner of the state of Wisconsin. I am now in the process of trying to collect reimbursement for expenses incurred for the allergy test that was supposed to be covered by my HMO. I am on the road to recovery and am determined to get the message out to these doctors and insurance companies.

We must take our health into our own hands, as no one else will do it for us.

### ELAINE GORDON

Elaine and I have been friends for more than 25 years, and she now lives next door to me in our condo complex. She is a mother of two, grandmother of five, and great grandmother of one. She is an intelligent, articulate person with good observational skills. Elaine was widowed several years ago and has picked up the pieces of her life by becoming active in organizations, both secular and religious. She maintains her figure by working out regularly at a gym. She is 5'3", wears a size 14 petite, and has allowed her once raven mane to become naturally gray.

### Elaine's Story

I've lived all my life with an irritable bowel. I was also one of those kids who got one cold after another. Other than that, I was pretty healthy until about 15 years ago.

At 55, I started getting disabling lower back pain. An MRI showed two slightly slipped discs, but the pain seemed out of proportion to this. I started reading books about the back and concluded that the discs weren't causing the problem, something else – maybe spastic muscles – was disturbing the discs. An orthopedist put me in bed with lots of anti-inflammatories that wreaked havoc with my stomach. Chiropractic treatment after the bed rest provided quite a bit of relief, but I was still in a lot of pain.

Claire is my next-door neighbor and Mah Jongg companion, and one day, somewhat facetiously, she said, "I'm tired of your problems ruining our Mah Jongg game." She suggested I see Dr. Sweeney, her internist.

Sweeney said I had muscle spasms, and suggested physical therapy. That helped, but I was still in pain, and once again Claire was the one who suggested that maybe I have fibromyalgia. I resisted, but when I thought about some of my symptoms – depression, sleeplessness, backache, irritable bowel, joint pains – I thought maybe I should consider it. I had the tender points, too. I thought I was just getting old and things hurt.

I was of two minds when I was diagnosed in 1994 at age 70. "For pity's sake, what else can go wrong?" part of me thought. But I also thought, "Maybe I can do something about this."

I wasn't too crazy about the idea of eliminating things from my diet. I had had bypass surgery in 1993 and already had enough diet restrictions, as far as I was concerned. ELISA/ACT™ found I was sensitive to cow dairy products, sulfites, celery, yeast, sodium benzoate (a preservative), boysenberry, caffeine, and rabbit. Actually, I remember eating rabbit once on a trip and suffering terrible backaches afterward.

I wasn't thrilled with all these limitations, but once I set my mind on something, I can do it. The yeast intolerance means no sugar, and I do like sweets. That was probably the hardest. But there was much more – if it comes in a bag, a bottle, a jar, or a can, I don't buy it anymore.

Four months after starting this restrictive diet, I began to feel better, and after six months, I felt great. I do cheat a little, but I've learned how much I can take. I don't hesitate to go anywhere or do anything. I don't concentrate on what I can't eat, I concentrate on what I can eat.

I don't know if I'll live longer with this diet, but I'll certainly enjoy life more.

---

Recently I had the opportunity to interview three more of the participants of the 1994 study. Le Trombetta, Mary Klaver and Kathy Woloczyk, all remain on the ELISA/ACT™ program.

**Le Trombetta** is on the road to health again thanks to the ELISA/ACT™ program. She has had three additional tests done since 1994. She is feeling somewhat better but still feels she has a long way to go. She has had two metabolic liver dysfunction tests that have revealed liver damage which, she was told, was initiated by prolonged use of acetaminophen prior to starting the ELISA/ACT™ program. She was also diagnosed with Lyme disease in 1994.

**Mary Klaver** is still on the ELISA/ACT™ program and doing well. She uses homeopathy and ayurveda-type alternative medical treatment to deal with underlying sources of problems unrelated to fibromyalgia. She attends a special water aerobics class offered at a local hospital.

**Kathy Woloczyk** continues to feel really good. The

ELISA/ACT™ program worked and made such a difference, she says, that, "It gave me back my life." A former self-proclaimed Junk Food Queen, she remembers what she felt like prior to May of 1994. Those memories serve as a reminder to do the right thing now. If she is off her diet for a lengthy period of time – 30 days – she knows the difference. She works out three times a week – 40 minutes each on the treadmill and weight training, and off and on does some yoga.

I was also fortunate to be able to interview some new ELISA/ACT™ participants.

**Jocelyn Standiford** didn't want to be on medications the rest of her life. She searched for a different way and determined that foods may be part of it, so the ELISA/ACT™ made sense to her. Her pain level was nine on a scale of one to ten – she couldn't run or play sports. Jocelyn has three children, and she wanted to be a mom and wife, and to socialize again. She feels very good now and has been on the ELISA/ACT™ program one and a half to two years. Six months into the program she was off all antidepressants. An unrelated mental problem has completely resolved itself, and she no longer is depressed, nor has intrusive thoughts or obsessive behaviors. Her pain, however, went up before it went down. Jocelyn had no support from the doctor who drew her blood for the test. She had to educate him. The hard part for her was getting started, finding information as well as the proper foods. Her main food culprit is beet sugar, and she can immediately tell the difference in body pain and in her brain functions. When she starts craving sugar, she uses Vitamin C in capsule form, and chromium.

**Rose** (who requested we not use her last name) has been on the ELISA/ACT™ program about one year. She had tried everything else, including medications from her rheumatologist, and then she researched delayed sensitivities. She does well when she sticks to her diet; when she doesn't, she has setbacks. The one thing she feels is out of her control is chemicals, which she feels she can't avoid 100%.

**Bonnie Kaprelian** heard about the ELISA/ACT™ from Kathy Woloczyk. She was tested in April/May of 1998. Her physician had pushed her to use rectal anti-inflammatories, which caused her to have diarrhea. Once she had the test, she knew better. Now she knows that when she stays away from her reactive items, she feels better.

# Chapter 16
# 1995: COMPLICATIONS

*Presence of mind and courage in distress
are more than armies to procure success.*
— DRYDEN. *AURENG-ZEBE.* ACT II, LAST LINES

In late November, several weeks after Joseph's 75th birthday, we settled uneasily in Florida. Personal tragedy loomed on the horizon. Along with the chaos of my restricted diet and the study, there were the usual routines of work, family, holidays, and travel. My husband and I were also coping with the rapid deterioration of the health of his daughter Randi, who had inflammatory breast cancer. It was a very sad time. She was diagnosed in May of 1993, and in the subsequent 20 months she was subjected to – as one oncologist described it, "slashing, burning and poisoning," – more commonly referred to as surgery, radiation, and chemotherapy. Finally in 1994, she underwent a bone marrow transplant.

Those 20 months were a roller coaster of mixed emotions. Each medical procedure was anticipated with high hopes and optimism, and each time the hopes were dashed with recurring symptoms.

Although doctors told Randi inflammatory breast cancer has a prognosis of six months to two years, we all yearned for the medical breakthrough that would change that outcome. She had two small children, 7 and 10, so each day was a precious opportunity to help them become more self-sufficient and independent. For Randi and her husband Keith, these were years of agony as they worked with the doctors to stamp out the brush fires of each increasingly damaging symptom of the spreading cancer.

We had reluctantly left Milwaukee with Randi's assurance that she would be okay. But, even though we had not braved a Milwaukee winter for years, our anxiety about her health tugged us home. We packed our bags, loaded up the car, and returned home the last week in December.

Randi died January 4, 1995. I couldn't help but be struck by the irony that I was obsessed with a project to help others to get better, but I could do nothing to help my stepdaughter. It was a tremendously frustrating feeling.

Less than seven short years prior, we had experienced one horrendous loss, and now here was another. Having learned how to get on with life after Pam's death, we mustered those skills once again.

Joseph and I talk to each other about our feelings of loss, and listened when our children wanted to share their feelings. We also had the attitude that we still have a life to live, and need to show our children that the joy, happiness, and pleasure of life can go on, even when tinged by our shared sadness.

Joseph and I stayed in Milwaukee for the customary 30 days of mourning according to Jewish tradition, and then we returned to Florida. Typically, it was the women who were the cement that held the extended family together. Since the loss of our two daughters, it takes more effort for us "women" to maintain the closeness with their families.

During this difficult month, I felt fatigue and an undercurrent of low-level pain. Chalking this up to the mental pain, I waited to see if the symptoms would diminish when we were back in Florida. To some degree they did, but there was a slightly nagging residual of underlying pain and more fatigue than I was used to.

By trial and experimentation, I have discovered some important things about this program of avoidance and repair. As I become healthier, I have learned I can indulge moderately in some of the items on my "forbidden" list. I am most likely to do this when dining away from home, and I always do it selectively. I may experience a low-level return of symptoms, but diligently watching my intake for 24 to 48 hours will usually return me to wellness.

That winter, however, I could not seem to shake the persistent low-level pain and fatigue. When these symptoms refused to disappear, despite careful attention to my food intake, I decided to take the ELISA/ACT™ test again.

I had the test readministered when I returned home in the spring. This time I was also tested for environmental chemicals, toxic minerals, and therapeutic foods.

To my surprise, I no longer showed a reaction to many of the items from the original list – perch/mackerel, cranberry, cherry, mango, cantaloupe, honeydew, venison, coffee, hops, tapioca, herbal teas, oysters, Brazil nuts, allspice/arrowroot, caraway seeds, vanilla, beet sugar, broccoli, white potatoes, garlic and organophosphate.

However, I now tested positive to tricholoethylene, maleic anhydride, aspartame, MSG, milk casein, coconut, corn, cola, malt, English walnut, black walnut oil, cinnamon, black-eyed peas, carrots, white and yellow onions, halogenated biocide, and bok choy.

Although the list appears shorter, there are complications with many of the items. When one is sensitive to two or more items in a particular group, all the items in the group must be avoided. Because aspartame and MSG are part of the additives and preservatives group, I needed to avoid all the other items in that group, which includes BHA, food coloring, saccharine, sodium benzoate, and, of course, sulfites. Casein is the basic protein in milk which, therefore, precludes the consumption of any dairy products.

Corn products have endless usage and are increasingly used in many of our processed and prepared foods and medications, in the form of cornstarch, food starch, and corn syrup. As more foods become fat-free, corn syrup is being added in greater quantities to make these foods palatable. In addition to the incredible number of prepared foods that contain corn, it is also found in stamp and envelope glues, chewing gum, and toothpaste.

I called the Crest toothpaste company to find out if their products, which I had been using, contain corn. I was told they do. I went to a health food store to find toothpaste that is free of both corn and coconut, since coconut was also on my list. Many toothpastes contain both of these items, but I did find one with neither – Pink Toothpaste with Myrrh. Myrrh, a spiced resin from Arabia, is used to maintain healthy gums. So is krameria, an astringent from Peru that is highly esteemed by the Andean Indians, who called it the gum root.

This toothpaste contains no detergent, no preservatives, no saccharine or sugar, no artificial colors, no chemical whiteners, and is available in health food stores. Since switching to this product, I no longer have bleeding gums.

It was interesting that I now had a sensitivity to corn. This came about in January of 1995, immediately after ethanol (a corn derivative) was added to the gasoline sold in Wisconsin. After this changeover, according to the local newspaper, many people in Wisconsin complained of flu-like symptoms. This relationship was dismissed by those in power who make these decisions.

Between the corn and the preservatives, I am in a precarious position where medications are concerned. My research suggests that almost all injected medications are preserved with sulfites. Just as I found that there is a sulfite-free Novocain, I hope other sulfite-free medications will be available to me if I ever need them. Pill forms of medication contain cornstarch as a binder, and items such as cough medications are sweetened with corn syrup. With my sensitivities, this makes it even more challenging to stay healthy.

Although I can now drink coffee and tea, I have been without these beverages for so long that I have no desire to reintroduce them into my diet. I drink only water – cold and hot. The heat of the beverage is satisfying for me and for others who have tried it at my suggestion. I do not have any particular food cravings. I feel healthy and have more energy than I remember having as a teenager, or as a young woman in my 20s and 30s.

From time to time, I have reflected on this and recall that I had food sensitivities at various times in my life. When I was a child, my mother tried to feed me a healthful diet. But, as kids are wont to do, I rebelled against her efforts and was a "picky" eater. She said I resisted milk, and would only drink it laced with chocolate syrup. Canned spaghetti with tomato sauce was a staple of my diet.

As a teenager, I adored butterscotch sundaes, even though I did feel a little queasy after eating them. When I ate a heavy meat and potatoes dinner, like the delicious stewed-beef dinner my mother cooked when I was in high school, I couldn't stay awake to do my homework. But then, I thought, who could?

One experience stands out vividly. I stayed overnight at the home of a high school friend, and in the evening we made ice cream sundaes with crushed pineapple topping. Now I know, of course, that preserved pineapple is packed with sulfites. Shortly after eating the sundae, I had severe gastric problems, and I fainted. In the morning, my friend's mother called a doctor. Those were the days when doctors made house calls. I had a stiff neck, aches and pains, extreme fatigue, but no fever. In the early 1950s, when this occurred, polio was a major concern.

The doctor suggested that I stay in bed for several days, and if no further symptoms developed, or I felt better, I could go home. After three days of their hospitality, I was somewhat recovered, and they politely suggested it was time to go home, a five-minute drive away.

Through the years, I had many adverse reactions to specific foods, but never made a connection between these responses and my overall health. And although I was seldom sick, I was a low-energy kid. I avoided, like the plague, active sports such as basketball or volleyball in gym class. Riding a bicycle was out of the question.

I recall that my mother, too, was always tired. She spent a lot of time resting on the sofa. She was 37 years old when I was born, and I just assumed it was because she was "old" when I was a teenager. She complained of chest pains when she vacuumed, and she rarely did anything strenuous. Ultimately she suffered congestive heart failure. I wonder now whether her fatigue and pain were symptoms of fibromyalgia, since her doctors never found any other serious medical problems.

At various other times in my life, I had difficulty with dairy products and bread items. It was not, however, until the 1980s, when I was overwhelmed by the convergence of a number of dietary changes – eating most of my meals in college cafeterias or restaurants, and the increase of additives and preservatives to many foods – that my system was so strongly impacted that it drove me to seek medical help.

---

I was also dealing with another medical mystery that eventually turned out to be related to the food and chemical sensitivities.

In September of 1993, two months after a trip Joseph and I had taken to the Middle East, my manicurist noticed a strange growth under my nails. She encouraged me to visit a dermatologist. His superficial diagnosis was a nail fungus, and he recommended treatment with an antifungal cream, Loprox. I used the cream during our stay in Florida that winter and watched the condition worsen. I went to a health food store and they recommended Tea Tree Oil, which was supposed to work miracles. It didn't.

When I returned to Milwaukee, I went to another dermatologist who, after listening to my explanation of my sensitivities, recommended the latest medical fad for fungus, Diflucan.

Fluconazole (the generic name for Diflucan) is used to treat severe fungal infections, such as mouth or esophageal fungus (thrush), systemic fungal infections, and other serious infections such as cryptococcal meningitis. I believe this drug should not be used to treat trivial fungal nail infections because of the possible side effect of serious liver damage.

Although I should have known better, I took it, because the doctor told me to. She prescribed 21 pills to be taken once a day for 21 days. The cost was over $200. The drug affected my sleep for the entire course of the treatment. Not because of the cost, but because of a sensitivity to the medication. For 21 nights I barely slept, and I walked around in a fog all day. When I stopped ingesting the Diflucan, the sleep problems went away immediately.

I next tried Sporonox, another antifungal, with no better results.

Then the dermatologist suggested I ingest 200,000 units daily of Vitamin A for two months, because she thought I might have a strange malady called Darier's Disease. After checking with Dr. Schwartz, I took 200,000 units of water-soluble Vitamin A daily for the next two months.

Meanwhile, I went to the Wisconsin Medical College Library to research this condition. Nowhere in the medical literature about Darier's Disease did I find mention of a nail fungus related to this condition. Rather, the descriptions talked about encrustation of the skin, somewhat like eczema, and brown papules (small inflammatory spots) on the skin.

When the Vitamin A treatment failed to produce any results, and my nails became more mottled and fragile, the female dermatologist referred me to the chief dermatologist at a local hospital.

His recommendation was also Loprox, the antifungal cream. However, a superficial biopsy of debris under the nails did not turn up fungus. He then suggested removing one of the nails for a more thorough biopsy. I declined his offer, since I would be leaving soon for Florida. When I told the doctor this, he referred me to a well-known "nail doctor" in Miami Beach. I continued to use the antifungal cream, and the mottling remained, but the debris disappeared.

My visit to the Miami Beach physician turned out to be an interesting experience. The nurse questioned me about my health history, and when I mentioned that I had had a basal cell carcinoma removed from my face a few years earlier, she suggested I visit the office regularly for a complete physical. I wasn't sure what a complete physical with a dermatologist entailed, so I asked for an explanation.

She said they would check my entire body for further carcinomas each time. When I told her that I am a snow bird – the Floridians' description of the winter residents – she dismissed me with, "Well, then you don't have to come." The Miami dermatologist asked me to hold out my hands so he could see my nails. He looked at them very briefly, from a distance, decided there was nothing there, said I should get a manicure and forget my nails, and billed my insurance company $100 for his words of wisdom.

I did what I was told. I had manicures and tried to forget my nails as I watched them separate from the nail beds. The condition worsened. In the summer of 1995, I returned, humbled, to the first dermatologist I had visited. As I explained what I had tried for the past two years he laughed and said, "Well, now we don't have to try those procedures."

He did offer me a small ray of hope. He shared with me

that when he was in medical school, a resident did research on a similar nail condition. The outcome was evidence of a sensitivity interaction between sunlight and nonsteroidal anti-inflammatory drugs. He suggested I use sunblock #30 on my fingers, just below the nails, and refrain from using NSAIDs. He prescribed an old-fashioned remedy (from the 1930s), c-Thymol in chloroform, which had to be prepared by a pharmacist – at a cost of $7.45 per month – to be applied under my nails three times a day. He told me it might take six to nine months for the nails to grow out.

When I returned to see him four months later, there had been tremendous improvement. The nails were gradually adhering to the nail beds and beginning to look healthy. Again, it had taken a lengthy search, but I had hit upon a solution to my problems. I have since learned that this remedy is very commonly used in Florida, but the solution is mixed with alcohol instead of chloroform.

This rather lengthy nail story highlights the problems that I perceive will haunt me in relation to any future medical problems I may have. If the problem is at all related to food or chemical sensitivities, there will be a lot of guesswork on the part of doctors to diagnose and treat it.

On my part, I am very concerned about my reactions to any and all medications and high doses of nutritional supplements. After my reaction to the Diflucan, I have become even more cautious about ingesting any medications. Because of its impact on the liver, for several months after ingesting the high doses of Vitamin A, I had trouble digesting foods with almost any kinds of fats – even olive oil. I needed to take digestive enzymes similar to Pepcid, prescribed by Dr. Schwartz, to alleviate the discomfort.

# Chapter 17
# 1996: Results To Take Us To The Future

*I firmly believe that if the whole <u>materia medica</u> could be sunk to the bottom of the sea, it would be all the better for mankind and all the worse for the fishes.*
— O. W. Holmes. Lecture. Harvard Medical School

In the Midwest winter struck hard and early. I was able to sit in the Florida sunshine and bask in the warmth as I read Patricia Deuster's report (complete with charts and graphs) on the results of our fibromyalgia study. I felt like celebrating when the report was finally in my hand, but as I read, my emotions were more complex than simple rejoicing. Having lived with this project, the study results were somewhat anticlimactic.

I could see that although the skirmish was over – I had proved there is a relationship between food and chemical sensitivities and the symptoms of fibromyalgia – my battle was just beginning. I had to get the word of hope out to those who suffer from fibromyalgia, and to the medical community who cares for them.

The report seemed fairly definitive to me. It outlined the staggering dimensions of the fibromyalgia problem. In the last decade as many as seven percent of patients who see family doctors or go to a general practice medical clinic describe fibromyalgia symptoms. A survey of young and middle-aged women in Norway found fibromyalgia in 10.5 percent of that population! The study used the diagnostic criteria developed by the American College of Rheumatology.

In describing the ELISA/ACT™ test, the report of the study noted that most healthy subjects will have two or less positive responses to the 300 or more substances tested, while people with fibromyalgia or other auto-immune or immune system dysfunctions will react to 10 to 50 of the substances. And the bottom line was this:

> Six months of avoiding sensitizing agents and taking nutritional supplements ameliorated many of the symptoms of fibromyalgia in the treatment group, whereas further decline or no improvement was noted in the control group.
>
> To be more specific, after six months, those with primary fibromyalgia experienced 50% less pain, 70% less depression, and 30% less morning stiffness than at the start of the study. Meanwhile, energy was elevated by 50%. But in the control group, after six months, reports of pain were higher, and depression was up 25%. The irritable bowel syndrome that so many of us suffer from also was decreased by 50% in the experimental group, compared to no changes in the control group. (Deuster 1996)

Dr. Deuster did point out some flaws in the study. First, it was not blinded; that is, the participants knew they were receiving the treatment that was being studied, and the control group knew they were not. It would be very difficult to blind a study like this one, where subjects follow an individualized protocol to eliminate a list of items from their diet and environment.

Also, the results depended upon the compliance of the participants, and that cannot be guaranteed. The people in the study were asked to make difficult – often radical – changes. As Dr. Deuster wrote, "Education, persistence, patience, commitment, and a willingness to change and go by the results are the prime requisites for this program to have its fullest expression."

But, this challenge was balanced by some of the results we observed. The study concluded:

> Some patients follow this treatment program and in six months report themselves to be completely free of fibromyalgia symptoms, despite having had fibromyalgia for 10 years or more and previously being a multiple treatment failure. (Deuster 1996)

I wanted to put a string of exclamations points after that sentence. *This treatment worked when nothing else did!*

Some portions of the study were of particular interest to me. It was fascinating to see the cluster of substances that resulted in the most reactions. I shouldn't have been surprised; many of them were precisely the substances that had plagued me for years.

From 20 to 42.5 percent of the study participants reacted

to MSG, Candida albicans (yeast), food colorings, caffeine, chocolate/cocoa, cola beverages, cow dairy products, xylene, sulfite/metabisulfites, yogurt, aspartame, BHA, cadmium, lead, acetaminophen, sodium benzoate, and oranges.

More than 22 percent of the study participants demonstrated a sensitivity to sulfites. Yet, the FDA has labeled sulfites "generally recognized as safe" because, according to their figures, less than five percent of the population is sensitive to this preservative.

In 1958, the FDA approved a Food Additives Amendment to the Federal Food, Drug, and Cosmetic Act of 1938, prohibiting the use of food additives until they had been proven safe. However, the law exempted substances "Generally Recognized As Safe" (GRAS), based on prolonged use and no compelling evidence of harmful effects. Sulfites were among those substances grandfathered onto the GRAS list, and thus never went through rigorous testing to study the occurrence of adverse health effects. Most recently, Congress abolished the GRAS list and directed the FDA to study the possible health benefits of healthy antioxidants and the health risks of immunotoxins (like sulfites).

While I understand that the people in the study who had fibromyalgia might be more sensitive than the general public, the testing of healthy subjects by the Serammune Physicians Lab has demonstrated that 14 percent of the general population may be sensitive to sulfites. I think this is something that bears further investigation by the agencies responsible for public health.

Another area of significance is the high frequency of environmental sensitivities diagnosed in the study participants. A number of medical researchers have observed the overlapping symptoms of patients with fibromyalgia, chronic fatigue syndrome, and multiple chemical sensitivities. Is it possible that these conditions are one and the same, with a range of symptoms that defy cut-and-dried diagnosis? Is it possible that a diagnosis of fibromyalgia, or CFS, or MCS, is related as much to the orientation of the diagnostician as it is to the syndrome itself?

This is an area that is ripe for intensive scientific inquiry. The compliance issue is, of course, a disturbing one. The ELISA/ACT™ program is not a magic bullet that will restore health in a matter of days or weeks. The evidence, however, is convincing that the nutritional changes can turn lives around if patient compliance is exercised, although it does not happen overnight.

The program, to be successful, requires a test of will along with a sincere desire to make necessary lifestyle changes. As Dr. Deuster noted in our study, "At least six months, and then perhaps even longer (depending on degree of compliance and on accuracy of laboratory assessment), are needed to help restore balance and function to a system that has been compromised for many years. However, this study clearly indicates that given a commitment, the ELISA/ACT™ program can be effective for sustained remission in many cases of fibromyalgia."

When we returned to Milwaukee, I sent a copy of the study results to each participant.

Several weeks later, I made some follow-up calls. From those who continued to comply with this program, I received responses ranging from, "Doing fine," to, "Feeling wonderful." Some participants still had underlying problems, such as digestive disorders, which still continue to be treated.

"Not doing very well," was the standard response from those who had stopped complying with the treatment requirements.

If there is one clear result from this study, it is that the questions it raised must be examined further, with the objectivity and rigor of any scientific investigation, so that we can get closer to results that are conclusive and incontrovertible.

A copy of the study authored by Patricia Deuster, Ph.D., M.P.H., entitled *A Novel Treatment for Fibromyalgia Improves Clinical Outcomes in a Community-Based Study*, is available, at no charge, to anyone interested, by calling the Serammune Physicians Lab at 1-800-553-5472.

## Chapter 18
## HOW CAN YOU BEGIN?

*Eat to live and not live to eat.*
— BENJAMIN FRANKLIN, POOR RICHARD, 1733

I have shared my story and experiences with you.

Now, having come to this point in the book, are you ready to consider food and chemical sensitivities as contributing factors to your symptoms of the mystery syndrome called fibromyalgia? Before you say yes, ask yourself the following questions:

- Have I exhausted all medical inquiry, including a complete blood chemistry screening, to rule out other conditions that might be afflicting me along with the fibromyalgia?
- Am I still looking for a magic pill for treating the symptoms of fibromyalgia?
- Am I willing to make permanent lifestyle changes, including modifying my eating habits and making exercise an integral part of my life?
- Will my family be helpful and cooperative in this endeavor?

- What will I need to do to overcome roadblocks to success?

This program requires the fullest participation, as well as your acceptance of the responsibility for its success. You need a high level of awareness of how you feel and what symptoms you are experiencing.

You need to know and understand the information that is available, to be informed, even if you disagree with the information. This will better enable you to communicate with your physicians. And most of all, you need the patience to accept that these might be long-term life-style changes.

Dr. Jaffe refers to this system as one of "defense and repair." My experience indicates a four-part program as follows:

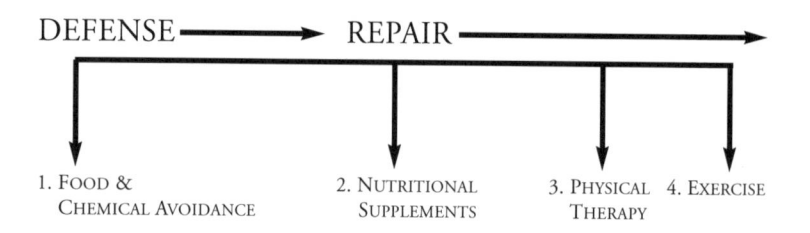

```
DEFENSE ─────▶ REPAIR ────────────────────▶
    │              │            │          │
    ▼              ▼            ▼          ▼
1. FOOD &      2. NUTRITIONAL  3. PHYSICAL  4. EXERCISE
CHEMICAL AVOIDANCE  SUPPLEMENTS   THERAPY
```

## 1. FOOD AND CHEMICAL AVOIDANCE (DEFENSE)

It is very difficult to correlate your own symptoms with exposure to common medications, foods and food additives, environmental chemicals, and toxins. The reactions may be delayed for hours or days. The ELISA/ACT™ is an excellent tool for pinpointing foods and chemicals that you are sensitive to. A comprehensive listing of the foods and chemicals tested by the ELISA/ACT™ is presented in Appendix A.

**Procedure for the ELISA/ACT™.** One ounce of blood is drawn to be used for a lymphocyte (white blood cell) culture.

The white cells are a common pathway for all delayed or hidden immune sensitivity reactions. The result of the test is a comprehensive, patient specific, fingerprint of immune responses.

From this information, a program of individualized recommendations – avoidance and/or substitution of reactive foods and chemicals – can be established.

There are two options for having the ELISA/ACT™ administered. You can call the Serammune Physicians Lab for information regarding insurance coverage, and for a referral to a physician in your area. Or, preferably, you can ask the physician who is now treating you for fibromyalgia if he or she is willing to arrange this test for you. Have your physician contact the Lab for information and for the kit for the blood-drawing procedure.

After you have completed the test, the lab will send your physician the results of the ELISA/ACT™ Lymphocyte Response Test indicating the intermediate and strong reactions (A copy of my results is presented in Appendix B); a list of recommended nutritional supplements; and a description of items tested, which will inform you about possibilities of exposure as well as substitutions for these toxic substances (Appendix C contains an example for Dairy Foods).

This material guided me on the road to health. It is also tremendously helpful to physicians who may not be totally knowledgeable about the world of nutrition and immunotoxins.

Since nothing else has worked, and you are probably as frustrated and discouraged as I was, perhaps in the interest of scientific inquiry your physician will agree to participate.

## 2. Nutritional Supplements (Repair)

The white blood cell culture together with a health appraisal questionnaire are used to determine an individual's nutritional supplement needs and necessary lifestyle changes. Again, this is an individualized program. In our study, however, the following supplements were used by all the treatment participants:

- Amino acid/Lipotropic combination – free radical, defense sulfur-containing amino acids to enhance detoxification; glycine; reduced glutathione; choline and inositol
- Multi-vitamin mineral preparation with transporters and cofactors
- Bio-Quercitin – blend of quercitin and OPC bioflavinoids
- Bone Guard – formulation of minerals, transporters, and cofactors needed by body for bone and joint health
- Mg PLUS – a blend of magnesium glycinate, ascorbate, citrate, and chloride
- Buffered Vitamin C – fully buffered ascorbate salts (calcium, magnesium, potassium and zinc)

From my own experience and observation, as well as feedback from study participants, I recommend introducing supplements gradually. Since it is likely that fibromyalgia patients have a hypersensitive immune system and may have unpredictable reactions to prescription medications and over-the-counter drugs, it is important to slowly introduce anything that is ingested. Take one supplement for a week, and if you do not perceive any unusual reaction (something you have not experienced before), add another until all have been introduced.

As you may recall from my story, I removed some identifiable foods from my diet while I was on vacation. Almost a month later, I started the nutritional supplements.

An interesting letter appeared in the "People's Pharmacy." The column, written by Pharmacists Joe and Theresa Graedon, appears in the *Sun Sentinel,* a local Florida newspaper.

> Dear People's Pharmacy:
>
> My father takes aspirin for his heart, Prednisone for arthritis, Zantac for heartburn and Hydralazine for high blood pressure. I wonder how all this medicine affects his vitamin levels. He complains that his feet tingle or feel numb, and he is not as sharp as he used to be.

In response to the letter, the pharmacists wrote:

> Many medications can deplete the body of crucial nutrients. Aspirin can keep Vitamin C from getting into cells. Prednisone [used for arthritis] leads to a loss of potassium and vitamins B-6, B-12, and folic acid. It also interferes with Vitamin D, which affects calcium metabolism. Zantac and other acid-suppressing drugs can make it difficult to absorb Vitamin B-12. And Hydralazine depletes B-6.
>
> When B vitamins, especially B-6 and B-12 are too low, the nervous system can suffer. Symptoms may include numbness and tingling of the hands and feet.

Your dad's mental decline may also be related to low Vitamin B-12 levels. His doctor should do a complete nutritional workup and recommend supplements."

Obviously, one must consider the side effects of long-term use of medications, particularly as they relate to nutritional supplement needs. It is also essential to purchase a high quality supplement. Not all supplement brands are created equal. The label must specify that the supplement does not contain any of the items to which you may be sensitive, such as wheat, corn, gluten, sugar, wax, soy, yeast, zein, sulfates, phosphates (other than coenzymes), preservatives, casein or other milk derivatives, or pectin (which contains sulfites). Also, be cautious of herbal remedies which may have an alcohol base. For maximum benefits, be prepared for long-term use of the supplements.

### 3. PHYSICAL THERAPY (REPAIR)

It is essential to have an Osteopath or Physical Therapist skilled in myofascial release as part of your treatment team. (See Chapter 12.) Before physical therapy can provide the maximum benefit, however, it is important to remove the toxins from the muscles by starting food and chemical avoidance. As the toxins are eliminated, the muscles become more pliant to the manipulations of the therapist.

You need a practitioner who will listen respectfully while you relate what you know about your own body. It is important for you to play an active role, helping your doctor help you and helping yourself get well.

Tell your doctor when a treatment procedure is working or when it is making you worse. Body awareness is a vital component in this process. As your body becomes more relaxed, you will become more aware of the tension when it occurs, providing a kind of feedback to enable you to consciously relax those muscles.

## 4. Exercise (Repair)

Caution! If you have not been exercising regularly, take four to six weeks on food and chemical avoidance (Defense) and nutritional supplements and physical therapy (the first two Repair segments) before introducing an exercise program. This will reduce or eliminate the microtrauma to your muscles.

Always consult your physician or physical therapist about the most suitable exercise program for you.

A good way to begin is to assess your pulse rate. To take your pulse, you will need a watch that can display seconds. First, find your pulse in your wrist or neck. Then count the beats within a 10-second period. Multiply that number by six to get your pulse rate per minute.

To determine your maximum desirable pulse rate at peak exertion, subtract your age from 220. Your goal should be to achieve a pulse rate of 80 percent of your maximum and to sustain this for at least 20 to 30 minutes, three to five times per week.

For example, my age, 65, subtracted from 220, is 155. Eighty percent of 155 is 124. My resting pulse rate is 60 to 66. Soon into my walk, I should reach a peak rate of near 124 and then sustain it for 20 to 30 minutes.

Start slowly. This avoids muscle microtrauma, small tears in the muscle caused by too strenuous exercise. You can gradually increase the challenge of your exercise program.

Remember, you are not entering a marathon, but introducing lifestyle changes that will benefit your health forever.

Always exercise on an empty stomach. Your body has enough work to do without having to digest food at the same time.

Never exercise until your muscles have been warmed up. Because muscles of fibromyalgia patients often feel tight and stiff, very gentle stretching of all major muscle groups for about five minutes before and after exercise will help reduce the chance of muscle injury. If you like to exercise first thing in the morning, take a warm or hot bath or shower beforehand. It may sound weird to bathe before exercising, but the benefits are amazing. Besides which, it will be some time in the future before you work up a sweat while exercising. Take my word on this, the outcome is wonderful.

## ADVANTAGES OF EXERCISE

- Exercise keeps muscles strong and flexible.
- Even mild aerobic exercise removes toxins from your body tissues and organs by increasing oxygen use.
- The Yoga Joint and Gland Exercises stimulate the internal organs to function more competently and efficiently to remove toxins. They can be done from a sitting position (on a chair) or standing.
- Exercise reduces stress and boosts endorphins which are proteins that decrease feelings of pain and increase a feeling of well-being.
- Exercise boosts the levels of serotonin – a chemical compound in the brain – that has a calming, stress-reducing effect and produces a state of feeling good.

- Long-term exercising results in stronger bones and a reduced possibility of osteoporosis later in life.
- Exercise helps with weight management. Building up to 30 minutes each exercise session, three to five times a week, is sufficient. It is not necessary to increase the time – better to increase the repetitions or the distance.

## Kinds of Exercise

**Walking.** Haven't exercised in a long time? Try walking. It is a surprisingly effective strategy for lifelong good health. Walking briskly can boost immune response and improve circulation. To begin a walking program, keep in mind that you're in no big hurry. This is lifetime health, not overnight magic. If you can only walk to the house next door and back, that's just fine. Each time you do this, add just a little more distance. Bad weather? Walk in a nearby shopping mall. Many malls open early for this purpose and even have medical personnel on hand periodically to test your heart rate, pulse, and blood pressure.

No fancy equipment is needed — only a good pair of walking shoes with a firm heel cup for stability, and plenty of room for toes so they can spread out as they push off. Wear loose comfortable clothes.

To make walking a habit takes willpower — and sometimes a strategy. Schedule regular walks with a friend, or walk first thing in the morning before other commitments. Vary your route to keep it interesting, or get a dog. Finally, don't think of it as exercise. It's time you've set aside for yourself. Enjoy it!

**Swimming or Water Aerobics.** The buoyancy of the water

makes movement easier. Many YMCAs, community centers, and health clubs have certified instructors to lead these programs. If you know how to swim, do laps. The purpose is not speed and distance, but the stretching effect of various strokes. Try the backstroke to stretch back muscles and expand the chest wall.

**Stretching.** Slow and easy range of motion stretches, which your physical therapist can recommend, are best. If there is any discomfort or pain, reduce the amount of stretch or the number of repetitions. In addition to the stretching exercises, strengthening exercises are beneficial and contribute to good posture and relief of lower back strain. These may include sit-ups, performed with knees bent, at the start of each stretching exercise program.

**Rebounding.** A rebounder, or mini-trampoline, can be used at home for short periods (minutes) with positive effects. Start with just a few minutes and increase a minute or two each week.

**Yoga Exercises.** Hatha Yoga can be done at a gentle level for beginners. I recommend Tape II of the Joint and Gland exercises which can be done sitting in a chair or on the floor. Abdominal breathing is also taught on this tape. At the end of both sides of the tape are wonderful relaxation exercises that can also be done sitting in a chair or lying on the floor. These exercises are very effective for stimulating your internal organs to work more effectively.

Another good exercise using rhythmic body movements is T'ai Chi Chuan, which combines gentle toning and graceful movements.

**Stationary bike.** Start with no resistance for no more than five minutes, if this exercise is new for you. Increase the resistance and time gradually, within your comfort zone. Don't force it.

**Treadmill or NordicTrack**™ for walking indoors. Start slowly and work up to a level that is comfortable for you. I have heard some people start with the treadmill and later add the arm movements on the NordicTrack.

**Weight Machines** such as Nautilus, where the weights can be adjusted. More repetitions can be performed at lower weights for arms, neck, shoulders, and back. It is especially important to be monitored by a doctor, exercise trainer, or physical therapist as the program progresses.

Don't make exercising difficult. Choose an exercise that you like to do and one that works best for you in terms of time, energy, and money. Whatever you select beats not exercising at all.

## Chapter 19
## MY LIFE TODAY

*To eat is human, to digest divine.*
— CHARLES L. COPELAND

At this point you may be wondering what my health is like today. At age 68, I am never fatigued and am rarely tired unless it is close to my bedtime of 11:30 P.M. to 12:00 midnight. I have no identified tender points and would not now qualify as a fibromyalgia patient.

Since 1992, I have had no recurrence of irritable bowel syndrome, anxiety, depression, itchy scalp, bleeding gums, photophobia, temporomandibular joint pain and thinning hair. My problems related to thinking and concentrating never returned after I obtained the full list of sulfited foods and eliminated them from my diet. My headaches ceased after I eliminated all dairy products.

*The Journal of Rheumatology* has a questionnaire for determining the severity of fibromyalgia by looking at one's ability to do the following: shopping, laundry with a washer and dryer, preparing meals, washing dishes and cooking utensils by hand, vacuuming a rug, making beds, visiting friends and relatives, yard work, and driving a car.

I do all of the above, and in addition, I entertain friends and family, and prepare brunches and dinners for six or eight guests.

Because Joseph is not fond of driving, I drove the entire 1,648 miles from Milwaukee to Florida this year, with only two overnight stops. I averaged 10 hours per day at the wheel. I chauffeur most of my friends because I believe my driving skills are better than theirs.

My typical day in Florida starts with a one-half-hour, two-plus-mile walk before breakfast, then the usual household chores, followed by four or five hours on my screened-in patio (with the balmy breezes wafting through) working on this book to let you know there is life and wellness after a diagnosis of fibromyalgia. But wait, the day is not yet over. There is dinner preparation and Mah Jongg with friends, or meeting friends for dinner, a movie, a play, or other activities. Occasionally, in the midst of all this, I will swim for 30 minutes when time and weather permit.

My day in Wisconsin is similar, with adjustments for the weather.

Out of curiosity, I had the ELISA/ACT™ test redone in 1997. My strong reactions were to nickel, malt, allspice/arrowroot, and cinnamon. The intermediate reactions were to chloroform, rhubarb, corn sugar, and the two major food groups of corn and berries. Although dairy was not indicated on the test, I still have a mild reaction, which causes some tissue swelling and retention of fluids, primarily in my thighs, hips, and hands.

Because I have made the avoidance of potentially toxic food and chemicals a long-term lifestyle change, I no longer have any desire to eat many of the items eliminated from my diet: coffee, tea, or bottled beverages; and chemically-treated meats containing nitrates, such as sausage, bologna, or hot dogs. I even feel somewhat repulsed when others eat these foods. The only time I feel sluggish or not 100 percent is when I push too far by consuming foods that contain even small amounts of dairy or corn several days in a row. I still limit my intake of sulfites by choosing not to eat processed, canned, or bottled foods, except when dining away from home.

When I have a desire to eat sweets, I increase my intake of Vitamin C, which quickly takes care of that craving. As a result, I have maintained my weight consistently for almost ten years without needing to curtail my appetite for those foods that appeal to me and those that I can eat in quantity. My most recent physical exam, in the spring of 2001, included a complete blood chemistry panel, showing all outcomes in the normal range.

Do I feel deprived? Sometimes. Do I feel healthy? Absolutely. Do I now have fibromyalgia? No! What I do have are food and chemical sensitivities that are under my control. I can choose those days and times when I want to challenge the limits of my tolerance to toxic exposure.

The author of a book I recently read suggested one should accept that fibromyalgia has become a part of your life and not focus too much on what makes you feel better or worse. He goes on to say that you should, therefore, accept the limitations of what has become "normal" for you.

This is not logical to me. If fibromyalgia is nondisabling and nondisfiguring, it seems to make more sense to find those physical and emotional activities that contribute to feeling better and those that create wellness. My philosophy is to consider all noninvasive and nontoxic possibilities, and to focus on correcting the problematic symptoms.

Reflecting on this whole experience of illness and my journey to wellness, I have come to some conclusions about the relationship between personal empowerment and health.

My reading and research have confirmed that the mind and the body are linked through the immune, endocrine, and central nervous systems. There appears to be no disease that is not mental and emotional as well as physical.

It was formerly believed that neuropeptides (chemical messengers) were located only in the brain and nerve tissue. Candace Pert, former chief brain biochemist of the National Institutes of Mental Health, and other researchers have found that these nervous system chemicals land on and activate receptor sites located in the body's endocrine and immune system cells, as well as in nerve cells. In addition, other body organs, including the kidney and bowel, also have receptor sites for these so-called "brain" chemicals. The actions of these chemicals directly influence the way in which thoughts and emotions affect our physical bodies.

We can set ourselves up for physical distress because of the biochemical effect of emotions on our immune and endocrine system. The immune system can be depressed by many of the symptoms associated with fibromyalgia: mental depression, fatigue, a sense of hopelessness and despair, and the inability to cope with even low levels of exposure to environmental and food-based chemicals. Many fibromyalgia patients can pinpoint a painful or traumatic event that seems to trigger the suppression of the immune system and the autoimmune response.

Given this relationship between the mind and the body, I

believe feelings of self-empowerment are essential in the healing process. While struggling to get a diagnosis and treatment for my symptoms, I developed a personal healthcare philosophy. I gave medical practitioners very few opportunities for guesswork. If a procedure was nontoxic and noninvasive, I stayed with it for a period of time. If there was no diagnosis, and the prescribed medication was worse than the symptom, I immediately moved on to another practitioner. I have a very low tolerance for being a guinea pig in the practice of medicine. If the test suggested was invasive and the doctor gave no sound reason for its performance, I passed on the procedure (i.e., a myelogram recommended by the orthopedist).

As it turned out, my reluctance may have saved my life. A myelogram is an x-ray study of the spinal cord enhanced visually by the injection of a dye. My ELISA/ACT™ test results indicated a sensitivity to food coloring. I don't know how my body would have responded to that test. I have asked several doctors if they test for chemical sensitivities before these procedures and was told, "Only if we are made aware of the problem in advance."

I was fortunate to have medical insurance that paid for most of the testing and visits to many of the different medical disciplines. When I was not insured, I paid out-of-pocket. For many participants in the study, uninsured treatments caused great financial hardship. By not having a perspective on their health, and by having too much faith in the medical system which was not helping them, they stayed with some practitioners too long or continued procedures that were counterproductive or even damaging.

Because of a lack of knowledge on fibromyalgia, some

doctors prescribed medications, such as Prozac, for the depression resulting from the long-term pain. From personal experience and stories shared within support groups, I've seen that those of us with fibromyalgia are also very sensitive to medications. A little goes a long way.

When the toxins are eliminated and the vitamins start the healing process, colds, aches and pains, and sleepless nights are less frequent.

We have, for too long, believed in the myth that the doctor knows more about our bodies than we do; that the "expert" can cure us. We give control of our health to experts who may not have current information, may be gender biased, and may be unable to diagnose if the tests performed do not show a definitive condition. Physicians, because of their own discomfort with uncertainty, order many standard medical tests, which is no help with fibromyalgia, since it cannot be diagnosed by these tests. Frequently, the testing results in misdiagnosis or non-effective treatments, which can even lead to additional health problems.

Drugs with toxic side effects and/or surgery are the modern medical preference for treatment of disease. That which is natural and nontoxic is often viewed as inferior.

Dr. Willliam Faber, of the Milwaukee Pain Clinic, practices reconstructive therapy by stimulating tissue growth. He says:

> Holistic methods have trouble gaining a foothold because there is not a lot of profit in them.
>
> You don't have any products to sell. Nonpatented and nonsurgical areas of technology are totally neglected because they are not big revenue producers, even

though they've been shown repeatedly to be more effective than surgical and pharmacological techniques.

Meanwhile the public is persuaded to spend billions of dollars on pain-killing drugs, not one of which does anything to fix the problem causing the pain. (The Milwaukee Journal 1992)

But, there are new ways to look at wellness and health maintenance that consider alternatives to drugs and surgery, such as dietary changes, vitamins, noninvasive therapies, and lifestyle changes, including moderate exercise.

We must accept responsibility for our own wellness and consciously determine to be a partner in our treatment. It is imperative that we schedule basic health-care tests, such as mammograms, pap smears, blood tests, cholesterol and blood pressure checks at appropriate intervals.

Moreover, it is important to have a doctor or health practitioner whose attitudes and beliefs about healing reflect our own ideas.

Grab the brass ring and discover your own journey to wellness. Your road may be fraught with bumps, detours, and blind curves. At these obstacles, call on your courage to persist, and even alter the route to your destination. I like to think that my formative years gave me the will to travel the byways as well as the main road.

For me, what could have been a life of illness and despair has become an exciting experience. I wrote this book to share my experience with you and your friends or family members who have fibromyalgia, and to encourage self-empowerment. It is my gift of hope to you.

# Epilogue
# 2001

I have made it a self-imposed duty at this stage in my life to fight the battle — to get the word out that there is hope for a cessation of the symptoms of fibromyalgia.

Two newspaper articles have fanned that determination.

When I read the first article, entitled "UW [*University of Wisconsin*] Doctor Finds Value in Fen-Phen," I was horrified.

> Daniel G. Malone, an associate professor of medicine, said he has been treating one new fibromyalgia patient a week with the drug combination [Fen-Phen]... Fen-Phen is a slang term for two drugs, fenfluramine and phentermine, which encourage the release and activity, respectively, of two nerve transmission substances in the brain, serotonin and dopamine. Malone said he continues to use Fen-Phen despite reports this summer [1997] from Mayo Clinic that found a connection between the drug combination and severe heart valve damage. So far, 82 such cases have been reported to the Food and Drug Administration, either by Mayo physicians or by others.

The drugs already were known to cause a potentially lethal condition called pulmonary hypertension in rare instances...

Malone said reaction among colleagues to his use of Fen-Phen to treat fibromyalgia ranged from benign acceptance "When you have nothing else to offer, why not?" to opposition "You shouldn't be doing this, you have no proof." He also emphasized that he has a long waiting list and no longer accepts new fibromyalgia patients.

As for the possible hazards, Malone said, "I just make darn sure that they [the patients] understand the increased risk of the two disorders [fibromyalgia vs. severe heart valve damage or pulmonary hypertension]. The question becomes 'What is the benefit you gain versus the risk'?" *(Milwaukee Journal Sentinel,* September 1997*)*

Is that the question, Dr. Malone — a choice between permanent heart damage and/or death, or the discomfort of nonfatal fibromyalgia?

On September 13, 1997, the Food and Drug Administration removed fenfluramine and phentermine, from the market for *any* medical use.

But fibromyalgia patients get desperate. When they get desperate enough...

[Dr. Jack] Kevorkian and Dr. Georges Reding, a retired psychiatrist, left the body of a Boston man, 42, at Huron Valley Hospital in Commerce Township. A note said the Massachusetts man suffered from fibromyalgia, a painful but nonfatal muscle disorder. (*Boynton Beach Sun Sentinel,* March 1998)

With this second article, it became clear to me how desperate some fibromyalgia patients can become.

After 30 years of research and inconclusive theories, there are only two areas of general agreement in the medical community: 1) Fibromyalgia is probably the result of many different causes or factors; and 2) Treatment will require looking beyond the traditional medical model, in which every medical problem is the result of an organic or biochemical cause.

Meanwhile, the desperate patients are left with pain, fatigue, and worst of all, the frustration of being told that if they find the right doctor, get their stress under control, and develop a positive attitude *maybe* they will feel better.

How long will it take for the general medical community to become aware of the relationship between food and chemicals, and health? Eleven years after my diagnosis, I am *still* asking.

I am constantly motivated to continue my mission by the fibromyalgia patients I meet when I speak to support groups, patients of health and therapy centers, and the general public. All of the people I have talked with agreed that the one thing they needed most was a support system. They wanted help getting started, they wanted to exchange information, share what they have learned about how to contact food processors and chemical companies, discuss reactions to vitamins and talk with those who have been on the program some length of time.

I want it for them, and for all of us.

While cruising through the Panama Canal in January of 1999, my husband Joseph and I serendipitously met Dr. Marshall Mandell. Dr. Mandell was working on a paper for a medical journal, regarding food and chemical sensitivities. We talked for an hour about his experiences and mine and about how difficult it was to convince the mainstream medical practitioners that the symptoms of medical problems might be related to allergic responses to food and chemicals.

I was elated to find that there are some medical practitioners who have been working on this concept for more than 40 years. Maybe we are closer to a major breakthrough in medical care than I had thought possible.

Several weeks after the cruise, I met with Dr. Mandell in his hometown of Bradenton, Florida. Before I departed, he generously gave me three of his books. I have shared with you some of the information they contain, which dovetails with my research. They answer the questions of how we have come to this point in medical history, and where decisions will have to be made on how to cope with the proliferation of autoimmune problems, which are presenting themselves not only to the older generations, but to children as well.

> Nature demands that what is taken out of the soil must be returned to it. Human health can't be any better than the quality of the food eaten. It is as simple as that. If the food has been chemically treated and processed, the quality of the food is changed. If the fruit and vegetables were grown in poor soil, the food has got to be deficient in vitamins, minerals, and trace elements.[1]

In 1979, when Dr. Mandell's book, *Dr. Mandell's 5-Day Allergy Relief System,* was published, the medical community was barely aware of a syndrome soon to be named fibromyalgia. With at least 5 percent of the population — 10 to 12 million people — now diagnosed and labeled with fibromyalgia, isn't it time for us to be concerned about the food we eat, the air we breathe, and the water we drink?

Shortly after the publication of his book *Food for Life,* in 1993, I attended a lecture on vegetarian eating by Neal Barnard, M.D. I chatted with him briefly about his lecture, explained why I couldn't eat some of the recommended foods because of my food sensitivities and we talked about fibromyalgia and my forthcoming study.

He has stayed in touch over the years and had sufficient faith in the outcome of my fibromyalgia study to inform his readers about what I had learned. He discusses the relationship between food and chemical sensitivities and fibromyalgia in his book, *Foods That Fight Pain,* published in 1998.

Dr. Barnard is president of the Physician's Committee for Responsible Medicine, a non-profit organization that promotes vegetarian eating and is known for rating airport food and school lunch programs.

He believes that certain foods can trigger pain while others ease pain, and emphasizes:
"We are just starting to recognize the power that food has."

Very little has changed in the past three years. I am encouraged to continue my mission to spread the word about fibromyalgia and wellness from an article in The New Yorker

[1] Mandell, Marshall, M.D., and Lynne Waller Scanlon. *Dr. Mandell's 5-Day Allergy Relief System.*

magazine November 13, 2000 entitled HURTING ALL OVER by Jerome Groopman, a physician.

In the era of managed care, doctors have neither the time nor the incentive to listen to a seemingly endless list of inexplicable symptoms. Fibromyalgia patients often set off a game of clinical hot potato, with each doctor eager to pass the patient on to a colleague as quickly as possible. One doctor referred to these patients as the "bane of the medical profession."

Thomas Edison said, "THE DOCTOR OF THE FUTURE WILL GIVE NO MEDICINE, BUT WILL INTEREST HIS PATIENTS IN THE CARE OF THE HUMAN FRAME, IN DIET, AND IN THE CAUSE AND PREVENTIONS OF DISEASE."

Let us hope we are on our journey in that direction.

# Appendices, Resources, & References

# Appendix A
## Comprehensive List of Items Tested

**Environmental Chemicals**
1.2 Dichlorobenzene
2,4 D
2,4,5 T
2-Methyl Pentane
3-Methyl Pentane
Acacia (Arabic Gum)
Aldrin
Benzaldhyde
Benzene
Benzo-pyrene
Benzyl Acetate
Beryllium Oxide
BHT (Butylated
 Hydroxytoluene)
Calcium Propionate
Carbon Disulfide
Carbon Tetrachloride
Carrageenan
Chlordane
Chloroform
Cis-dichloroethylene
 cyclohexylamine
DBCP (1,2-dibromo-3
 chloro-propane)
DDT
DEET (N,N-Diethyl-M-
 toluamide
Diacetyl (2,3 butanedione)
Dibutyl Phthalate
Dieldrin
Endrin
Ethyl Acetate

Ethyl Acetoacetate
Ethyl Butyrate
Ethylene Dibromide
Gelatin
Heptachlor
Hexachlorocyclohexane
Hydrolyzed Veg. Protein
Isopropylether
Latex:
 Polystyrene, Styrene
 Divinylbenzene
Malleic Anhydride
Methoxychlor
Methylene Chloride
Morpholine
Nitrosamine Mix
Pentachlorophenol
Phthalates (Phthalide)
Pinene
Polysorbate 60
Polysorbate 80
Potassium Bromate
Propyl Gallate
Propylene Glycol
 (1,2 propanediol)
Pyrene
Selenium Sulfide
Silicates (Silicon Dioxide)
Silicone
 [Poly (Dimethylsiloxane)]
Sodium Benzoate
Sodium Fluoride
Sodium Propionate

Sorbitol
Tert-butyl-ethyl Ether
Tert-butyl-methyl Ether
Tetrachloroethylene
Toluene
Tragacanth
Trichloroethylene
Vinyl Chloride
Xylene
Xylitol

**Toxic Minerals**
Aluminum
Arsenic
Cadmium
Lead
Mercury
Nickel (II) Chloride

**Chemical Compounds**
Aldehyde/Formaldehyde
Detergent (Synthetic)
Metallic Catalysts (Ni)
Petroleum By-Products (Solvents)
Phenol
PWM (Poke Weed Mitogen)
Soap (SDS)

**Pesticides:**
Carbamates
Halogenated Biocide
Organophosphate

**Nutritional ELISA/ACT™ Additives & Preservatives**
Aspartame
BHA
Food Coloring
MSG (Glutamate)
Saccharine
Sodium Benzoate
Sulfite/Metabisulfite

**Crustaceans**
Crab
Lobster
Shrimp
Mollusks:
    Clam, Oyster, Scallop

**Dairy**
Butter:
    Clarified, Whole
Cheese (Cow):
    Brick, Cottage,
    Hard/Parmesan, Processed

**Milk:**
Casein
Cow Milk:
    Pasturized, Raw
Goat Milk (Incl. Cheese)
Sheep Cheese (Romano)
Yogurt

## Fish
Anchovy
Bass
Catfish
Codfish
Haddock
Perch/Mackerel
Red Snapper
Salmon/Lox
Sardine
Sole/Flounder/Halibut
Swordfish
Trout
Tuna
Turbot/Whitefish

## Fowl
Chicken
Goose/Duck
Turkey

## Fruit
Apple
Apricot
Banana
Blackberry
Blueberry
Boysenberry
Cantaloupe
Cherry
Coconut
Cranberry
Currant
Date
Fig
Grapes:
    Concord, Green, Red, White
Grapefruit
Honeydew
Kiwi
Lemon
Lime
Mango
Mandarin Orange
Nectarine
Orange
Papaya
Peach
Pear
Pineapple
Plum/Prune
Raspberry
Strawberry
Tamarind
Tangerine
Watermelon

## Grains
Amaranth
Barley
Buckwheat/Kasha
Corn (Maize)
Gliadin
Gluten
Kamut
Millet
Oats
Rice:
    Brown, White
Rye
Triticale
Wheat

## Meats
Beef/Veal
Chicken
Deer/Venison
Lamb/Mutton
Pork/Bacon/Ham
Rabbit

## Miscellaneous
Algae (Spirulina)
Aspirin/Coal Tar
Baker's Yeast
Baking Powder
Baking Soda
Brewer's Yeast
Candida Albicans
Caffeine
Chamomile
Chocolate/Cocoa
Coffee (Decaf. & Reg.)
Cola
Gin (Juniper Berries)
Hops
Kelp (Sea Weed)
Malt
Nitrates
Psyllium Seed
Rose Hips
Tapioca
Tea (black)
Tobacco
Tofu/Miso
Tylenol (Acetaminophen)

## Oils
Cod Liver
Corn
Cottonseed
Grapeseed
Hazelnut
Hydrogenated (Hardened Fat)
Linseed
Olive
Peanut
Primrose
Rape Seed (Canola)
Safflower
Sesame
Soybean
Sunflower
Walnut Oil (Black)

## Nuts & Seeds
Alfalfa
Almond
Anise Seed
Brazil Nut
Cashew
Chestnut
Hazelnut/Filbert
Macadamia
Peanut
Pecan/Pine
Pistachio
Poppy Seed
Pumpkin
Sesame
Sunflower
Walnut (English)

## Spices & Seasonings
Allspice/Arrowroot
Bay Leaf
Caraway seed
Cinnamon
Clove
Curry
Dill
Ginger
Horseradish
Mace
Nutmeg
Oregano
Paprika
Parsley
Pepper:
    Black, Cayenne, Chili, White
Peppermint
Rosemary
Sage/Basil
Spearmint
Thyme
Vanilla

### Sugars:
Beet
Cane
Corn
Honey
Maple
Molasses
Sucanat

## Vegetables
Artichoke
Asparagus
Avocado
Beans:
    Green, String, Wax
Beets
Black-eyed Peas
Broccoli
Brussels Sprouts
Cabbage
Carob
Carrots
Cauliflower
Celery
Chive
Corn
Cucumbers
Garbanzo (Chick Peas)
Garlic
Kidney Beans
Lentils:
    Green, Red
Lettuce:
    Endive, Iceberg, Red Leaf, Romaine
Lima Beans
Mushrooms
Navy/Ninji Bean
Olive
Peas:
    Green, Snow
Pimento
Pinto (Frijole)
Radish
Rhubarb
Rutabaga
Soya Bean
Spinach
Squash
Sweet Potato

Turnip (Incl. Greens)
Watercress
Yam

**Nightshade:**
Eggplant
Pepper:
    Green, Red, Yellow
Potato:
    White
Tomato

**Onion:**
Chive
Garlic
Leek
Parsnip
White/Yellow

## Therapeutic Foods
Astragulus
Bok Choi
Chinese Tea
Cucumber:
    Japanese, Sea
Dahlia Flower (Lectin)
Dashi Kombu
Dong Quai
Dried Laver
Eel
Elk
Ginseng:
    Chinese, Siberian, Other
Hijiki
Kombu (Lectin)
Miso:
    Barley, Brown, Hatcho, White, Yellow
Mushroom:
    Shiitake, Straw, Woodear
Oboro Kombu
Peony Flower (Lectin)
Plum (Umeboshi)
Quail
Red Oil
Resin
Royal Jelly
Snake:
    Rattle, Water
Tamari
Turtle
Wakame
Yaki Nori (roasted)

# Appendix B
## ELISA/ACT™ Lymphocyte Response Tests (complete)

ELISA/ACT™ Lymphocyte Response Tests (Complete)

Patient: Claire Musickant        Doctor: Norman Schwartz MD
Interpreter: _____        Phlebotomy Date: 6/19/95

A STRONG reaction is marked in the dot to the left of the item's number, and an INTERMEDIATE is marked to the right.

**Toxic Minerals**
- O T1 O Mercury
- O T2 O Lead
- O T3 O Cadmium
- O T4 O Nickel (II) Chloride
- O T5 O Aluminum
- O T6 O Arsenic
- O T7 O Control
- O T8 O Control

**Environmental Chemicals**
- O E1 O Control
- O E2 O Gelatin
- O E3 O 2-methyl Pentane
- O E4 O 3-methyl Pentane
- O E5 O Benzene
- O E6 O Toluene
- O E7 O Xylene
- O E8 O Cis-dichloroethylene
- O E9 O Ethylene Dibromide
- O E10 O Methylene Chloride
- O E11 O Pentachlorophenol
- O E12 ● Trichloroethylene
- O E13 O Vinyl Chloride
- O E14 O DBCP(1,2-dibromo-3 chloro-Propane)
- O E15 O Chloroform
- O E16 O Carbon Tetrachloride
- O E17 O Phthalates (Phthalide)
- O E18 O Dibutyl Phthalate
- O E19 O Silicone(Poly(Dimethylsiloxane)]
- O E20 O Research
- O E21 O Latex (Linked Polystyrene)
- ● E22 O Maleic Anhydride
- O E23 O Diacetyl (2,3-butanedione)
- O E24 O Potassium Bromate
- O E25 O Propylene Glycol(1,2Propanediol)
- O E26 O Silicates (Silicon Dioxide)
- O E27 O Tragacanth
- O E28 O Carrageenan
- O E29 O Hydrolyzed Veg. Protein
- O E30 O BHT

**Nutritional**
**Additives & Preservatives**
- ● 1 O Aspartame
- O 2 O BHA
- O 3 O Food Coloring
- O 4 ● MSG (Glutamate)
- O 5 O Saccharine
- O 6 O Sodium Benzoate
- O 7 O Sulfite/Metabisulfite

**Crustaceans**
- O 8 O Crab
- O 9 O Lobster
- O 10 O Shrimp

**Dairy**
- O 11 O Butter (Whole)
- O 12 O Butter (Clarified)
- **Cheese (Cow):**
- O 13 O Brick
- O 14 O Cottage Cheese
- O 15 O Parmesan
- O 16 O Processed Cheese
- O 17 O Research
- **Milk:**
- O 18 ● Casein
- O 19 O Cow Milk (Pasteurized)
- ● 20 O Cow Milk (Raw)
- O 21 O Goat Milk (Incl. Cheese)
- Soy (See 188)
- O 22 O Yogurt
- O 23 O Sheep Cheese (Romano)

**Fish**
- O 24 O Anchovy
- O 25 O Bass
- O 26 O Catfish
- O 27 O Codfish
- O 28 O Haddock
- O 29 O Perch/Mackerel
- O 30 O Red Snapper
- O 31 O Salmon/Lox
- O 32 O Sardine
- O 33 O Research
- O 34 O Sole/Flounder/Halibut
- O 35 O Swordfish
- O 36 O Trout
- O 37 O Tuna
- O 38 O Turbot/Whitefish
- O 39 O Research

**Fowl**
- O 40 O Egg White (Chicken)
- O 41 O Egg Yolk (Chicken)
- O 42 O Chicken
- O 43 O Goose/Duck
- O 44 O Turkey
- O 45 O Research

**Fruit**
- O 46 O Apple
- O 47 O Apricot
- O 48 O Banana
- **Berries:**
- O 49 O Blackberry
- O 50 O Blueberry
- O 51 O Boysenberry
- O 52 O Cranberry
- O 53 O Raspberry
- O 54 O Strawberry
- O 55 O Cherry
- ● 56 O Coconut
- O 57 O Currant
- O 58 O Date
- O 59 O Fig
- O 60 O Red Grape (Concord)
- O 61 O White Grape (Green)
- O 62 O Grapefruit
- O 63 O Kiwi
- O 64 O Lemon
- O 65 O Lime
- O 66 O Mandarin Orange/Tangerine
- O 67 O Mango
- O 68 O Cantaloupe/Honeydew
- O 69 O Watermelon
- O 70 O Nectarine

# Appendix B
## ELISA/ACT™ Lymphocyte Response Tests (complete)

Patient: Claire Musickant

| | | | | | | | | |
|---|---|---|---|---|---|---|---|---|
| O | 71 | O Orange | O | 113 | O Tea (Herbal) | O | 154 | O Ginger |
| O | 72 | O Papaya | O | 114 | O Tobacco (See 204-207) | O | 155 | O Horseradish |
| O | 73 | O Peach | O | 115 | O Tofu / Miso | O | 156 | O Mace |
| O | 74 | O Pear | O | 116 | O Tylenol (Acetaminophen) | O | 157 | O Mustard (Spice, Greens) |
| O | 75 | O Pineapple | O | 117 | O Yeast (Baker's) | O | 158 | O Nutmeg |
| O | 76 | O Plum/Prune | O | 118 | O Yeast (Brewer's) | O | 159 | O Oregano |
| O | 77 | O Tamarind | **Mollusks** | | | O | 160 | O Paprika |
| **Grains** | | | O | 119 | O Clam | O | 161 | O Black Pepper |
| O | 78 | O Amaranth | O | 120 | O Oyster | O | 162 | O Cayenne (See 204-207) |
| O | 79 | O Barley | O | 121 | O Scallop | O | 163 | O White Pepper |
| O | 80 | O Buckwheat/Kasha | **Oils** | | | O | 164 | O Peppermint |
| O | 81 | ● Corn (Maize) | O | 122 | O Cod Liver | O | 165 | O Rosemary |
| O | 82 | O Millet | O | 123 | O Cottonseed | O | 166 | O Sage/Basil |
| O | 83 | O Oats | O | 124 | O Grapeseed Oil | O | 167 | O Spearmint |
| O | 84 | O Rice (White) | O | 125 | O Hydrogenated Oil | O | 168 | O Thyme |
| O | 85 | O Rice (Brown) | O | 126 | O Linseed | O | 169 | O Vanilla |
| O | 86 | O Rye | O | 127 | O Primrose | **Sugars** | | |
| O | 87 | O Triticale | O | 128 | O Safflower | O | 170 | O Sucanat |
| O | 88 | O Wheat | O | 129 | O Rape Seed (Canola) | O | 171 | O Beet |
| O | 89 | O Kamut | **Nuts And Seeds** | | | O | 172 | O Cane |
| **Meat** | | | O | 130 | O Alfalfa | O | 173 | O Corn |
| O | 90 | O Beef/Veal | O | 131 | O Almond | O | 174 | O Honey |
| O | 91 | O Lamb/Mutton | O | 132 | O Anise Seed | O | 175 | O Maple |
| O | 92 | O Pork/Bacon/Ham | O | 133 | O Brazil Nut | O | 176 | O Molasses |
| O | 93 | O Deer/Venison | O | 134 | O Cashew | **Vegetables** | | |
| O | 94 | O Rabbit | O | 135 | O Chestnut | O | 177 | O Artichoke |
| **Miscellaneous** | | | O | 136 | O Hazelnut/Filbert | O | 178 | O Asparagus |
| O | 95 | O Algae (Spirulina) | O | 137 | O Macadamia | O | 179 | O Avocado |
| O | 96 | O Aspirin / Coal Tar | O | 138 | O Peanut | O | 180 | ● Black-eyed Peas |
| O | 97 | O Baking Powder | O | 139 | O Pecan/Pine | O | 181 | O Carob |
| O | 98 | O Baking Soda | O | 140 | O Pistachio | O | 182 | O Garbanzo (Chick Pea) |
| O | 99 | O Candida Albicans | O | 141 | O Poppy Seed | O | 183 | O Kidney Bean |
| O | 100 | O Caffeine | O | 142 | O Pumpkin | O | 184 | O Lima Bean |
| O | 101 | O Chocolate/Cocoa | O | 143 | O Sesame | O | 185 | O Navy/Ninji |
| O | 102 | O Coffee (Decaf. & Reg.) | O | 144 | O Sunflower | O | 186 | O Pea (Green/Snow) |
| O | 103 | ● Cola | O | 145 | ● Walnut (English) | O | 187 | O Pinto/Frijole |
| O | 104 | O Gin (Juniper Berries) | ● | 146 | O Walnut Oil (Black) | O | 188 | O Soya Bean |
| O | 105 | O Hops | **Spices & Seasonings** | | | O | 189 | O String/Wax Bean |
| O | 106 | O Kelp/Sea Weed | O | 147 | O Allspice/Arrowroot | O | 190 | O Beet |
| ● | 107 | O Malt | O | 148 | O Bay Leaf | O | 191 | O Broccoli |
| O | 108 | O Nitrates | O | 149 | O Caraway Seed | O | 192 | O Brussel Sprouts |
| O | 109 | O Psyllium Seed | ● | 150 | O Cinnamon | O | 193 | O Cabbage |
| O | 110 | O Rose Hips | O | 151 | O Clove | O | 194 | ● Carrot |
| O | 111 | O Tapioca | O | 152 | O Curry | O | 195 | O Cauliflower |
| O | 112 | O Tea (Black) | O | 153 | O Dill | O | 196 | O Celery |

# Appendix B
## ELISA/ACT™ Lymphocyte Response Tests (complete)

Patient: Claire Musickant

| | | |
|---|---|---|
| O 197 O Cucumber | **Chemical Compounds** | O 250 O Ginseng, Other |
| O 198 O Lentils (Green & Red) | O 225 O Aldehyde/Formaldehyde | O 251 O Ginseng, Siberian |
| O 199 O Endive | O 226 O Detergent (Synthetic) | O 252 O Chinese Tea |
| O 200 O Iceberg | O 227 O Metallic Catalysts (Ni) | O 253 O Research |
| O 201 O Red Leaf | **Pesticides:** | O 254 O Miso, Barley |
| O 202 O Romaine | O 228 O Carbamates | O 255 O Miso, Brown |
| O 203 O Mushroom | O 229 O Organophosphate | O 256 O Miso, Hatcho |
| **Nightshade:** | O 230 ● Halogenated Biocide | O 257 O Miso, White |
| O 204 O Eggplant | **Other chemicals** | O 258 O Miso, Yellow |
| O 205 O Bell Pepper | O 231 O Phenol | O 259 O Mushroom, Shiitake |
| (Green, Red, Yellow) | O 232 O Petroleum By-products | O 260 O Mushroom, Straw |
| O 206 O Potato (White) | (Solvents) | O 261 O Mushroom, Wood Ear |
| O 207 O Tomato | O 233 O Salicylate | O 262 O Research |
| | O 234 O Research | O 263 O Dahlia Flower (Cultorum) |
| O 208 O Olive | O 235 O Soap (SDS) | O 264 O Plum, Umeboshi |
| O 209 O Chive | O 236 O Research | O 265 O Quail |
| O 210 O Garlic | **Controls** | O 266 O Red Oil |
| O 211 O Leek | O 237 O Control | O 267 O Resin |
| ● 212 O White/Yellow | O 238 O Control | O 268 O Royal Jelly |
| O 213 O Parsley | O 239 O Control | O 269 O Dashi Kombu |
| O 214 O Parsnip | O 240 O Control | O 270 O Sea Cucumber |
| O 215 O Chili (Red) | | O 271 O Hijiki |
| O 216 O Pimento | **Therapeutic Foods** | O 272 O Yaki Nori (Roasted) |
| O 217 O Sweet Potato/Yam | O 241 O Peony Flower Parts | O 273 O Wakame |
| O 218 O Radish | O 242 O Astragulus | O 274 O Dried Laver |
| O 219 O Rhubarb | O 243 O Research | O 275 O Kombu |
| O 220 O Rutabaga | O 244 ● Bok Choi | O 276 O Oboro Kombu |
| O 221 O Spinach | O 245 O Cucumber, Japanese | O 277 O Snake (Rattle) |
| O 222 O Squash | O 246 O Dong Quai | O 278 O Snake (Water) |
| O 223 O Turnip (Incl. Greens) | O 247 O Eel | O 279 O Tamari |
| O 224 O Watercress | O 248 O Elk | O 280 O Turtle |
| | O 249 O Ginseng, Chinese | |

**"Let food be your medicine"**

Hippocrates

# Appendix C
## Description of Items Tested: Dairy Foods

**Dairy Items 11-23**

With the exception of clarified butter, and casein, the individual items in the dairy category should be familiar and self-explanatory. Occasionally people who think they react to dairy products actually are sensitive to thickeners like tragacanth and carrageenan or to corn.

If you are reactive to one or more products in the dairy family, especially if the reactive items include casein or cow milk (pasteurized or raw), it will be listed on your results as Dairy. We do this to draw your attention to the greater possibility of cross-reactivities in this group. We, therefore, recommend that you avoid all cow dairy products and substitute as described below. Avoid non-dairy substitutes as they often contain dairy fractions to which you may react. In particular, nondairy creamers usually have cow-milk antigens in them and should be avoided if you are cow-milk sensitive. (Examples include Cool Whip, Coffee Mate, Irish Cream, Mocha Mix and Lady Lee brand nondairy creamer.)

**Clarified Butter**

How would you like to use a cooking fat that does not bubble or smoke, contains no additives yet does not turn rancid and is nutritious? If so, become acquainted with ghee or clarified butter. Ghee is a derivative of butter made by melting butter down and removing all the milk solids. Ghee is available at many fine health food stores including from Purity Farms, Poolesville, MD.

## Casein

Milk protein can be disguised on package labeling as:

- casein, caseinate or sodium caseinate, whey or whey solids
- lactalbumin, lactoglobulin, or natural flavoring

Casein is milk protein. It can be hidden in a number of products not commonly thought to contain milk protein such as hot dogs, canned tuna fish, soy cheeses, breads, non-dairy creamers, butter substitutes, some sorbets, and others. In fact, it has been found in many products labeled as "nondairy". This misleading labeling has been of great concern to the medical community because it has resulted in severe allergic reactions in unsuspecting individuals with known dairy allergies.

### Foods that usually contain dairy (milk)

| Baked Goods | Sweets | Misc. | More Misc. |
| --- | --- | --- | --- |
| bread | candy | cheese | whey |
| rolls | ice cream | yogurt | hot dogs |
| biscuits | chocolate | margarine | canned tuna |
| crackers | | quiche | mashed potatoes |
| cookies | | creamed vegetables | soy cheeses |
| cakes | | creamed soups | nondairy creamer |
| pies | | white sauces | butter substitutes |
| | | sour cream | luncheon meats |
| | | cream cheese | salad dressings |

Milk products provide texture and a rich flavor, and are sometimes used to bind sauces or custards. Substitutions are relatively easy. Instead of milk or cream in a baked recipe, try water, fruit juice, or even vegetable soup stock, which is especially good in breads. In sauces, the most common substitution is sautéed pureed onions, carrots and/or turnips. Nut milk can be made by blending water with cashews or almonds in a two-to-one ratio, then straining. While the first thought may not be appealing, nut milk is quite tasty. In addition to its uses in cooking, it can be poured over cereal or enjoyed as a beverage.

When recipes call for ricotta cheese, cottage cheese, yogurt or sour cream, tofu is an excellent substitute. Crumble firm tofu and season it with a dash of soy sauce, and you have dairyless ricotta or cottage cheese. Blend soft tofu with a small amount of water and a teaspoon of lemon juice, and you have dairyless yogurt or sour cream. It is more difficult to substitute for hard cheeses, select Romano (sheep) cheese or goat cheese where possible and use "yeast cheese". Yeast cheese is based on nutritional yeast, a yellow, flaky powder that smells like chicken soup mix. Sold in health food stores, this yeast is grown on molasses, not on beer as in brewer's yeast.

# Appendix D
## Symptoms or Conditions

Fibromyalgia patients may also experience some of the following symptoms or conditions:

- Food sensitivities
- Chemical sensitivities
- Irritable bladder
- Irritable bowel
- Migraine headaches
- Feelings of swelling in hands and/or feet
- Hair loss
- Lethargy
- Micro-trauma to muscles
- Tension headaches
- Dizziness
- Mouth lesions
- Anxiety
- Depression
- Temperomandibular jaw pain
- Mental confusion
- Memory loss
- Concentration problems
- Trouble remembering words
- Cold hands and feet
- Nocturnal myoclonus
- Sleep disturbances
- Numbness and tingling in hands and feet
- Photophobia
- PMS
- Skin discoloration
- Scalp itch
- Body stiffness
- Eye problems such as pain or vision changes

# Resources and References

## RESOURCES

**The People's Pharmacy**
Write to:
Joe and Teresa Graedon
235 E 45th Street
New York, NY 10017
pharmacy@mindspring.com

**Fibromyalgia Network**
P.O. Box 31750
Tucson, AZ 85751-1750
1-800-853-2929
1-520-290-5508
FAX: 1-520-290-5550

Publishes the *Fibromyalgia Network,* a quarterly newsletter. The Network provides names of fibromyalgia-aware physicians by geographical area, as well as other resources.

**ELISA/ACT Biotechnologies, Inc.**
**(Serammune Physicians Lab)**
14 Pidgeon Hill Drive
Suite 300
Sterling, VA 20165
1-800-553-5472

**NoMSG**
P.O. Box 367
Santa Fe, NM 87504
1-800-BEAT-MSG (1-800-232-8674)
www.nomsg.com

**The Himalayan Publishers**
To order, or to request a free mail-order catalog, call or write:
RR1, Box 400
Honesdale, PA 18431
1-800-822-4547

## REFERENCES

Backstrom, Gayle, Dr. Bernard R. Rubin. *When Muscle Pain Won't Go Away.* Dallas, TX: Taylor Publishing Company, 1992.

Barnard, Neal D. *Foods That Fight Pain.* New York: Harmony Books, a division of Crown Publishers, 1998.

Bennett, Robert M. *Fibromyalgia (Fibrositis).* Third Edition: Arthritis Foundation, 1989.

Bennett, Robert M. "Chapter 33 – Fibrositis," *Textbook of Rheumatology.* W.B. Saunders Company, 1989.

Bennett, Robert M., Sharon R. Clark, Linn Goldberg, Donna R. Nelson, Peter Bonafede, John Porter, and David Specht. "Aerobic Fitness in Patients With Fibrositis," *Arthritis and Rheumatism* Vol. 32, No. 4. (April, 1989)

Bennett, Robert M., Sharon R. Clark, Stephan M. Campbell, Shirley B. Ingram, Carol S. Burckhardt, Donna L. Nelson, and John M. Porter. "Symptoms of Raynaud's Syndrome in Patients with Fibromyalgia," *Arthritis and Rheumatism* Vol. 34, No. 3. (March, 1991)

Birnie, Derk J., Alex A. Knipping, Martin H. van Rijswijk, Alida C. de Blecourt, and Niels de Voogd. "Psychological Aspects of Fibromyalgia Compared with Chronic and Nonchronic Pain," *The Journal of Rheumatology* 18:12. (1991)

Block, Sidney R., M.D. "Fibrositis and the Concept of Generalized Rheumatism: The Confessions of an Unrepentant Lumper," *Occupational Problems in Medical Practice*. Medical Publications, Inc., 1990.

Boissevain, Michael D., and Glenn A. McCain. "Toward an Integrated Understanding of Fibromyalgia Syndrome: Medical and Pathophysiological Aspects," parts 1 and 2, *Elsevier Science Publishers* B.V., 1991.

Brief Reports on Fibromyalgia and Psychic Distress, Fibromyalgia and Viral Infections, Fibromyalgia and Depression and Anxiety. (n.p., n.d.)

Briones, Esperanza, and Dwight R. Robinson. "Chapter 34 – Nutrition and Rheumatic Diseases," *Textbook of Rheumatology*. W.B. Saunders Company, 1989.

Bruce, Debra Fulghum, and Harris H. McIlvain, M.D. *The Fibromyalgia Handbook*. New York: Henry Holt and Company, Inc., 1996.

Bruckheim. Allan, M.D. "Low Doses Of Drugs Can Revive

Rheumatic Disorder," *Milwaukee Journal*, 1988.

Carette, Simon, Glenn A. McCain, and David A. Bell. "Evaluation of Amitriptyline in Primary Fibrositis," *Arthritis and Rheumatism* Vol. 29, No. 5. (May, 1986)

"Chronic Muscle Pain Syndrome," *Mayo Clinic Health Letter.* (January, 1991)

Crook, William G., M.D., *The Yeast Connection.* Jackson, TN: Professional Books, 1986.

Donovan, Patrick M., M.D., "The ELISA/ACT™ Test – Part 1: Its Role in Identifying Time-Delayed Reactive Environmental Toxicants," *Townsend Letter.* May, 1991 #94; June, 1991 #95.

Deuster, Patricia, Ph.D., M.P.H. *A Novel Treatment for Fibromyalgia Improves Clinical Outcomes in a Community-Based Study.* Serammune Physicians Lab, 1996.

Dunkin, Mary Anne, "Fibromyalgia: Out of the Closet," *Arthritis Today.* (September-October, 1993)

Ediger, Beth, "Coping with Fibromyalgia (Fibrositis)," Third Printing: *LRH Publications.* September, 1992.

"ELISA/ACT™ Clinical Update 12," *Serammune Physicians Lab* Volume 3, Number 3. (Fall 1994)

*Fibromyalgia Syndrome (FMS) – A Patient's Guide.* Fibromyalgia Network.

Freundlich, Bruce, M.D., and Lawrence J. Leventhal, M.D. "Comment on the 1990 American College of Rheumatology Criteria for Fibromyalgia," *Arthritis and Rheumatism* Vol. 33, No. 12. (December, 1990)

Goldenberg, Don L. "Fibromyalgia and Other Chronic Fatigue Syndromes: Is There Evidence for Chronic Viral Disease?" *Seminars in Arthritis and Rheumatism* Vol. 18, No. 2. (November, 1988): pp. 111-120.

Goldenberg, Don L. "Diagnostic and Therapeutic Challenges of Fibromyalgia," *Hospital Practice.* (September 30, 1989)

Goldenberg, Don L., David T. Felson, and Hal Dinerman. "A Randomized, Controlled Trial of Amitriptyline and Naproxen in the Treatment of Patients with Fibromyalgia," *Arthritis and Rheumatism* Vol. 29, No. 11. (November, 1986)

Goldenberg, Donald, M.D. "Fibromyalgia and Chronic Fatigue Syndrome," Lecture presented at Columbia Hospital. 8 June 1992.

Griffith, H. Winter, M.D. *Complete Guide to Symptoms, Illness and Surgery.* The Body Press, 1985.

Hench, P. Kahler, M.D. *Fibromyalgia – The Great Impostor.* AIMPLUS. (n.d.)

Jaffe, Russell, M.D., Ph.D. *Immune Defense and Repair Systems in Biologic Medicine I: Autoimmunity. Clinical Relevance of Biological Modifiers in Diagnosis, Treatment and Testing.*

Jaffe, Russell. Interview by Claire Musickant. Tape recording. Reston, Virginia, July 1996.

Klein, Linda "Fibromyalgia Syndrome: Shedding Light on the "Mystery Disease," *Arthritis Today.* (May-June, 1989)

Lue, Frank. "Sleep Studies," *Fibromyalgia Network.* (July 1993)

Lyme Disease Center at Robert Wood Johnson Medical School. "Lyme Disease and Fibromyalgia," *The American Journal of Medicine* Vol. 88. (June, 1990)

Mandell, Marshall, M.D., and Lynne Waller Scanlon. *Dr. Mandell's 5-Day Allergy Relief System.* New York, New York Harper & Row Publishers, 1979.

McCain, Glenn A., et. al. *Primary Fibromyalgia and Cardiovascular Fitness.* (n.p., n.d.)

Moldofsky, Harvey, Paul Saskin, and Franklin A. Lue. "Sleep and Symptoms in Fibrositis Syndrome after a Febrile Illness," *The Journal of Rheumatology* 15:11. (1988)

*No MSG.* Santa Fe, New Mexico. NoMSG, 1999.

Northrup, Christiane, M.D. *Women's Bodies, Women's Wisdom.* Bantam Books, 1994.

Reilly, Paul A. and Geoffrey O. Littlejohn. "Peripheral Arthralgic Presentation of Fibrositis/Fibromyalgia Syndrome," *The Journal of Rheumatology* 19:2. (1992)

Rice, Jon R., M.D. "Fibrositis Syndrome," *Medical Clinics of North America.* Vol. 70, No. 2. (March, 1986)

Russell, I. John, M.D., Ph.D. *Fibrositis/Fibromyalgia Syndrome.* The Clinical and Scientific Basis of M.E./CFS, 1994.

Schwartz, Norman. Interview by Claire Musickant. Tape Recording. Milwaukee, Wisconsin. July 1996.

Sigal, Leonard. *Arthritis Today.* (May - June 1993): pp.8.

Smythe, Hugh A., Aviv Gladman, Pierre Dagenais, Majed Kraishi, and Richard Blake. "Relation Between Fibrositic and Control Site Tenderness: Effects of Colorimeter Scale Length and Footplate Size," *The Journal of Rheumatology* 19:2. (1992)

Stedman, Thomas Lathrop. *Stedman's Medical Dictionary: Illustrated in Color (26th Ed.)* Lippincott, Willimas, and Wilkins, 1995.

Strauss, Steven, M.D. "FMS and CMS," *Fibromyalgia Network.* (July 1993)

Williamson, Miryam Ehrlich. *Fibromyalgia: A Comprehensive Approach.* New York: Walker and Company, 1995.

Wolfe, Frederick, M.D. "Fibromyalgia in the Elderly: Differential Diagnosis and Treatment," *Geriatrics* Vol. 43, No. 6. (June, 1988)

Wolfe, Frederick, M.D. *Fibrositis, Fibromyalgia, and Musculoskeletal Disease: The Current Status of the Fibrositis Syndrome.* (n.p., n.d.)

Yunus, Muhammad B., Fibromyalgia Syndrome: New Research on an Old Malady. 1989. (n.p.)

Yunus, Muhammad, Alfonse T. Masi, John J. Calabro, Kenneth Miller, and Seth L. Feigenbaum. "Primary Fibromyalgia (Fibrositis): Clinical Study of 50 Patients with Matched Normal Controls," *Seminars in Arthritis and Rheumatism* Vol. 11, No. 1. (August, 1981)

# ORDER FORM

## FIBROMYALGIA:
### MY JOURNEY TO WELLNESS

To order copies of *Fibromyalgia: My Journey To Wellness*, please complete the form below. (Please feel free to duplicate this form.)

I would like to order _____ copies of *Fibromyalgia: My Journey To Wellness* at $17.95 per copy (plus postage and handling).

**Book Total**
( _____ copies at $17.95 per copy)     $_____

**Sales Tax**
(Wisconsin Residents add $1.00)     $_____

**Shipping and Handling**
($3.50 for each book ordererd)     $_____

**Total Amount Enclosed**     $_____

**Ordered By:**
Name: _____
Address: _____
City: _____
State: _____ Zip: _____
Phone Number: (_____) _____

**Ship To (if different from above):**
Name: _____
Address: _____
City: _____
State: _____ Zip: _____

Please complete this order form and mail along with check or money order to:

Claire Musickant, P.O. Box 240035, Milwaukee, WI 53224
E-mail: cmusickant@aol.com

*10% of all proceeds are donated to the Health Studies Collegium for further Fibromyalgia Research.*